THE PSORIASIS DIET COOKBOOK

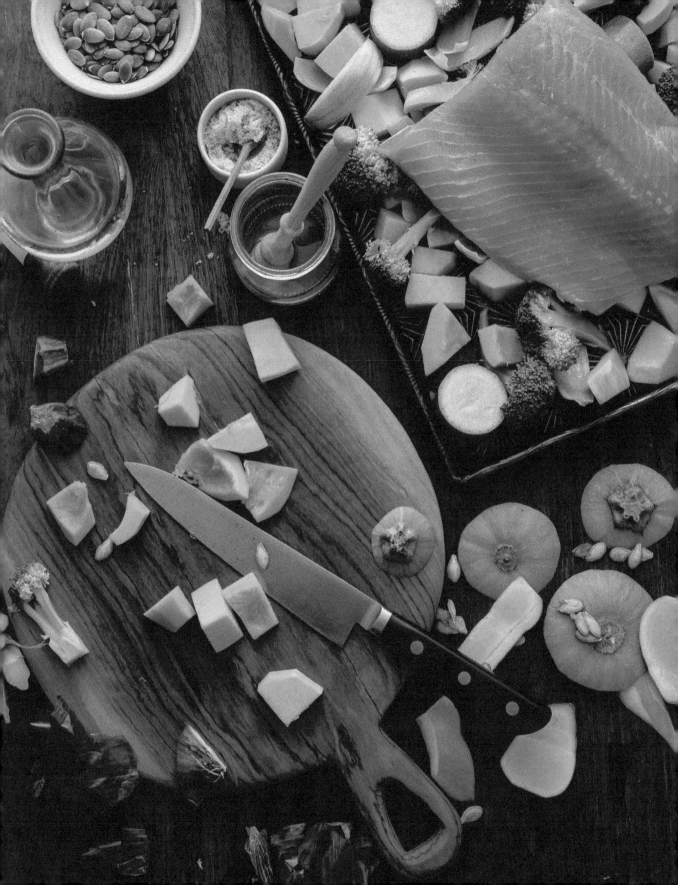

The Psoriasis
DIET COOKBOOK

Easy, Healthy Recipes
to Soothe Your Symptoms

KELLIE BLAKE, RDN, LD, IFNCP

ROCKRIDGE
PRESS

For general information on our other products and services or to obtain technical support, please contact our Customer Care Department within the United States at (866) 744-2665, or outside the United States at (510) 253-0500.

Rockridge Press publishes its books in a variety of electronic and print formats. Some content that appears in print may not be available in electronic books, and vice versa.

TRADEMARKS: Rockridge Press and the Rockridge Press logo are trademarks or registered trademarks of Callisto Media Inc. and/or its affiliates, in the United States and other countries, and may not be used without written permission. All other trademarks are the property of their respective owners. Rockridge Press is not associated with any product or vendor mentioned in this book.

Interior and Cover Designer: Darren Samuel
Art Producer: Sue Bischofberger
Editor: Seth Schwartz
Associate Editor: Samantha Holland
Production Editor: Sigi Nacson

Photography © 2020 Annie Martin. Food styling by Michael De La Torre.
Author photo courtesy of Kimmy Gillmeister.

ISBN: Print 978-1-64611-154-1 | eBook 978-1-64611-155-8

R0

To my IRONMAN husband, Will, who has changed everything about his life to join me on my healing journey. And to anyone navigating life with an autoimmune disease—there is always hope.

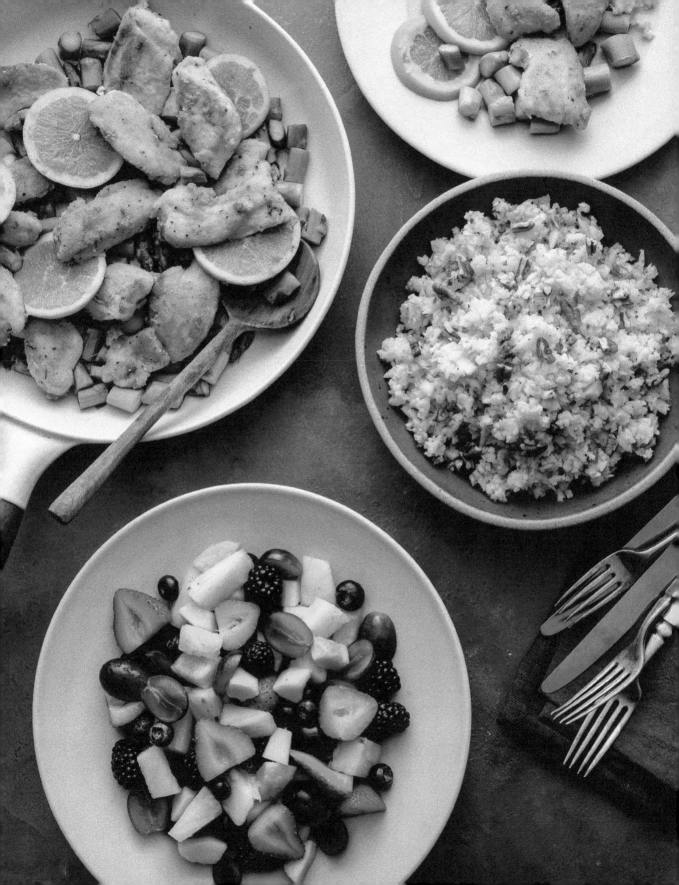

Contents

Introduction

I've had psoriasis for as long as I can remember. I didn't officially get diagnosed until my early teen years, but I first noticed symptoms around the age of five. I experienced psoriasis plaques on my scalp for the majority of my youth, then developed areas on the back and side of my neck in my early twenties. My sister also battled this disease, but her plaques were larger and located in more visible areas, such as her elbows, knees, and shins. We were both treated by a dermatologist with tar shampoos and topical steroids, and my sister also tried topical vitamin D and light therapy, all with minimal success. We both followed the standard American diet, and nutrition and lifestyle changes were never offered as treatment options.

My skin psoriasis has actually been in remission since my mid-twenties, but around that time I began experiencing other troubling symptoms. I fought Epstein-Barr virus and Raynaud's phenomenon and then noticed unexplained mouth sores, digestive distress, headaches, muscle aches, joint pain, lower back pain, sleep disturbances, swollen joints, and extreme fatigue. I experienced at least one of these symptoms every single day.

I sought conventional medical treatment from my primary care provider and was referred to several specialists in rheumatology, podiatry, and dermatology. I had several expensive tests and was diagnosed with everything from sleep deprivation to fibromyalgia to mild psoriatic arthritis, but none of the specialists could agree on anything definitive. I was prescribed numerous steroids and medications, all of which caused intolerable side effects. The one medication that seemed to make my symptoms bearable was a nonsteroidal anti-inflammatory drug (NSAID). NSAIDs are designed to be used for the temporary relief of pain and inflammation, but I remained on this class of drug for eight continuous years.

My breaking point came in 2017, when I began to suffer from severe digestive distress with all food intake and had to nap in my car on my lunch break because of excessive fatigue. I remember the last visit to my rheumatologist in May 2017, where I complained of unbearable symptoms. He simply said, "I have nothing else to offer you." I left his office deflated, hopeless, and almost at the point of tears. He was telling me I would just have to live with these symptoms for the rest of my life, which is a scary prospect for a young, active person. I desperately wanted to feel better and get back to my normal life, but seemingly no one could help me.

So I began to learn about functional medicine and functional nutrition. With encouragement from my cousin, Jaclyn Ruble, and my sister, Dr. Heather Skeens, I made some changes to my diet, added some nutritional supplements and essential oils, and began to practice yoga. My symptoms began to improve almost immediately, but I still struggled with fatigue. In November 2017, I visited the Cleveland Clinic Center for Functional Medicine and my life was forever changed. I learned the root causes of my symptoms and how to use lifestyle- and nutrition-related changes to reverse my symptoms and maximize my quality of life. After just nine months of functional medicine and nutrition, I was able to discontinue use of the NSAID medication (which I realized was actually contributing to some of my symptoms).

Psoriasis is a complex disease, and although my story is more involved than I can share in this short introduction, it's important to remember that nutrition and lifestyle factors can be used as the foundation for healing. Although there are some great conventional treatment options for psoriasis, including medications, vitamin D, and light therapy, this book will teach you how to add nutrition therapy as a way to improve your most debilitating psoriasis symptoms. These easy-to-make, delicious, anti-inflammatory recipes will be a valuable tool in your toolbox for preventing, and even reversing, the progression of your chronic disease!

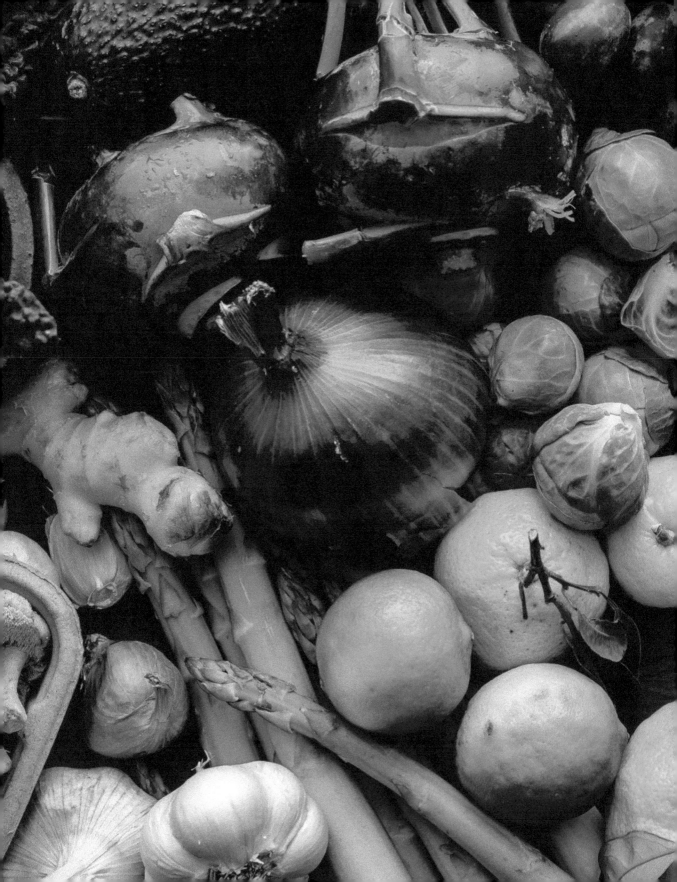

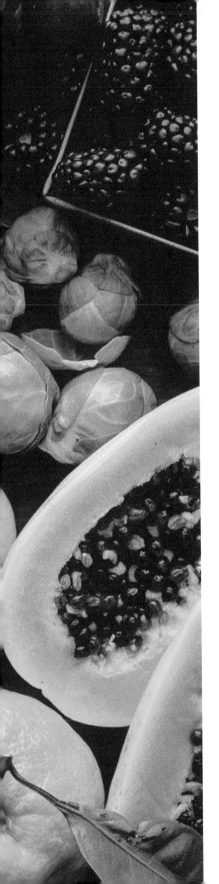

1
PSORIASIS AND DIET

Psoriasis is a chronic, T-cell–mediated autoimmune skin disease affecting up to 4 percent of the worldwide population. The outward signs of psoriatic disease are lesions on the skin that can range from mild to severe, but psoriasis can also affect the body systemically through an inflammatory process that increases the likelihood of serious chronic disease development. Some other diseases associated with psoriasis include metabolic syndrome, cardiovascular disease, type 2 diabetes, high blood pressure, fatty liver disease, depression, and inflammatory bowel disease. In addition to skin symptoms, 30 percent of those with psoriasis will develop joint pain in the form of psoriatic arthritis, which can become debilitating over time.

Genetic factors and environmental factors, such as chronic stress, exposure to toxins and smoke, infections, drugs, alcohol, and nutrition are likely responsible for the development of psoriasis.

A diet high in processed and refined foods, sugar, and unhealthy fats has been shown to contribute to and exacerbate symptoms of chronic diseases like psoriasis. By contrast, an anti-inflammatory diet high in plant-based foods and healthy sources of fat can reduce the risk of chronic disease and even promote symptom reversal. As with most autoimmune diseases, psoriasis symptoms occur in a cycle: they worsen, then they get better, only to reappear and worsen again, and so on.

Conventional treatment typically focuses on managing psoriasis symptoms, but nutrition-related changes—including following an anti-inflammatory diet—are quickly becoming a desired treatment to address the root causes of psoriasis.

EATING FOR HEALTH

Chronic diseases now affect six in ten Americans, and autoimmune diseases like psoriasis are rapidly increasing. There is debate about how autoimmune diseases originate. Although there may be many root causes, food is one important factor to consider. Certain foods can create an environment in the body that facilitates chronic disease development by triggering the inflammatory process. Inflammation can be a wonderful thing when you are trying to recover from an acute injury, but chronic, uncontrolled inflammation damages the tissues of the body and leads to disease. Think of inflammation as a smoldering fire. When there is a constant supply of fuel, the fire can grow out of control. Foods that inappropriately trigger the immune system can be one source of fuel for inflammation.

The immune system, most of which lives in the gastrointestinal tract, is designed to protect the body from toxins and organisms in the environment. Normally, when the body is under attack, the immune system mounts a healthy defense and prevents these foreign invaders from causing illness or disease. However, when chronic inflammation is present, as is the case in diseases like psoriasis, the lining of the gastrointestinal tract becomes compromised. Toxic substances that are meant to exit the body cross the intestinal barrier and get into the bloodstream and surrounding tissues. This confuses the body and causes the immune system to attack everything indiscriminately, even the body's own tissues, leading to symptoms of chronic disease.

The standard American diet—which is high in refined, processed, and gluten-containing foods; dairy products; unhealthy fats; and sugar—is known to increase the inflammation and symptoms of chronic disease. Restoring gut health by replacing triggering foods with nourishing anti-inflammatory foods is the place to start when healing diseases like psoriasis.

It has been said that you can't exercise your way out of a bad diet, but you can certainly cook your way out of a chronic disease. It is never too late to use nutrition-related strategies to minimize the potency of psoriasis symptoms. No matter how long you've suffered with psoriasis, you can always make changes that will begin to reverse the disease's progress and allow your body to heal. Although no specific diet or nutrient will cure psoriasis, an anti-inflammatory meal plan can provide the nutrients needed to quiet inflammation, improve the health of the gastrointestinal tract, and normalize the immune response. Powerful symptom relief is achievable, and it starts in the kitchen.

An anti-inflammatory diet is based on maximizing real, whole, delicious foods and minimizing the intake of trigger foods. Focusing your diet around vegetables, fruits, beans, and legumes provides a valuable anti-inflammatory benefit. In addition, the fiber found in these plant-based foods serves to improve your overall gut health. Fish, nuts, seeds, avocados, and olives provide powerful anti-inflammatory omega-3 fatty acids and mono-unsaturated fats. Good quality animal products, herbs, spices, and green tea also work to further reduce inflammation and allow for disease reversal.

LIFESTYLE HABITS THAT REDUCE INFLAMMATION

To experience the greatest benefit from the psoriasis diet, maintain an overall healthy lifestyle by incorporating these self-care techniques:

Manage stress in a healthy way. Unmanaged stress is an independent risk factor for chronic disease and reduces your quality of life. Although we can't avoid all the negative stress in our lives, we can learn healthy stress management techniques. Maintain healthy personal relationships and consider practicing meditation and yoga, which have been shown to reduce pro-inflammatory cytokines in the body and improve psoriasis symptoms, as well as reduce your body's stress response.

Maintain a healthy sleep schedule. Aim for 7 to 8 hours of sleep each night. Try to maintain the same sleep and wake times each day.

Exercise. Move your body in mindful ways to help reduce inflammation. Aim for at least 30 minutes of movement five days per week and add some strength training at least twice per week. Better yet, practice high-intensity interval training (HIIT) for even more benefit.

Quit smoking and avoid alcohol. Smoking increases inflammation in the body, and heavy alcohol use has been shown to increase the severity of psoriasis flares. In addition, both smoking and alcohol use can disrupt your body's sleep patterns.

Consider having a blood test to check your vitamin D level. Vitamin D is a hormone important in immune and inflammation control. Inadequate vitamin D is a common characteristic of chronic diseases that often occurs in association with psoriasis, and people with psoriasis typically have lower vitamin D levels. If your vitamin D level is low or inadequate, consider speaking with your doctor about supplementation methods.

FOLLOWING THE PSORIASIS DIET

Although there is no one perfect eating style that will cure psoriasis, an anti-inflammatory diet like the Mediterranean diet has been shown to reduce psoriasis severity and even prevent the disease.

The Mediterranean Diet

The Mediterranean diet has long been researched as a way to fight inflammation in the body and is used not only for disease prevention, but also as a form of medical nutrition therapy for many conditions, including rheumatoid arthritis, cardiovascular disease, diabetes, cancer, depression, obesity, and cognitive decline. This plant-based diet is high in fruits, vegetables, legumes, whole grains, fish, nuts, and extra-virgin olive oil while being low in eggs, meat, dairy products, and alcohol. The Mediterranean diet focuses on real food, is easy to implement, and addresses the root causes of inflammation by emphasizing healthy monounsaturated fats, dietary fiber, antioxidants, and polyphenols.

The meal plan provided in this book is a modified version of the Mediterranean diet. Psoriasis is an autoimmune condition, so avoiding gluten, dairy, and alcohol are key because all have been shown to exacerbate psoriasis symptoms. In addition, some people with psoriasis will need to avoid eggs and nightshade vegetables—potatoes, tomatoes, eggplant, and bell peppers are some of the most common—as both are known to have a pro-inflammatory effect.

Psoriasis Diet Guidelines

Eat routine meals and avoid refined carbohydrates. People with psoriasis are at risk of metabolic syndrome, a cluster of symptoms including high waist circumference, elevated triglyceride and fasting glucose levels, high blood pressure, and low "good" cholesterol levels. Psoriasis also brings an increased risk of type 2 diabetes, and high blood sugar has been shown to worsen psoriasis flares. Maintaining a routine eating pattern is a great way to stabilize blood sugar levels and can improve how you feel. Eat roughly the same amount of food at roughly the same times each day. During the day, try to go no longer than five hours between meals. Blood sugar levels are also significantly impacted by processed and simple carbohydrates. Although you will want to avoid foods with gluten altogether, it can also be helpful to limit some gluten-free grains, white rice, and processed sugar.

Choose anti-inflammatory and nutrient-dense foods at every meal. The majority of your plate should contain plant-based foods such as vegetables (especially leafy greens), nuts, seeds, and beans. Remember to include a source of healthy fat and some protein at each meal and use anti-inflammatory herbs and spices liberally.

Avoid inflammatory foods. Processed foods, gluten, dairy, sugar, processed red meats, eggs, unhealthy fats, and nightshades can all cause inflammation in the body. Some of these foods, such as eggs and nightshades, are actually nutrient-dense, but people with psoriasis and other autoimmune conditions may still need to avoid them, at least until the gastrointestinal tract is healed and the gut is healthy. If you are sensitive to nightshades and eggs, substitutes are provided in the recipes in this book.

Eliminate any food allergens and sensitive foods. True food allergies always need to be avoided, but sensitive foods can also create negative symptoms. When you consume sensitive foods, the inflammatory response is triggered, leading to psoriasis flares and other undesirable symptoms. Food sensitivities can change over time, so pay close attention to your symptoms to help determine which foods cause an adverse reaction. If a food bothers you, do your best to avoid it.

Allow three hours between your dinner meal and bedtime. Digestion requires a lot of energy. Giving your body time to process your last meal before bed will improve sleep quality and allow for rest and repair.

FERMENTED FOODS AND INFLAMMATION

The gut microbiome is a hot topic these days, and for good reason. We have trillions of bacteria in our gastrointestinal tracts that are responsible for many things, including creating vitamins and maintaining a healthy immune response. However, when those healthy bacteria are not in balance, toxic substances can cross the intestinal barrier, causing an increase in negative symptoms such as chronic fatigue, headaches, skin disorders, bloating, indigestion, diarrhea, constipation, brain fog, depression, and muscle and joint pain. An imbalanced gut microbiome is common in all autoimmune diseases, including psoriasis.

Modifying your diet and working to adopt an overall healthy lifestyle will help improve the health of your gut microbiome; moreover, adding fermented foods to your daily routine will enhance those effects.

Fermented foods are produced when microorganisms convert the carbohydrate in a food to lactic acid. Fermentation is not only a great way to preserve foods, but also creates beneficial probiotics to support a healthy gut microbiome. According to a 2019 review in *Nutrients*, fermented foods can improve digestive function, enhance the immune system, and allow for improved nutrient absorption. In addition, fermented foods can be used in combination with an overall healthy diet to lower blood pressure, blood sugar, and cholesterol. Fermented foods also improve the gut-brain connection and can help alleviate symptoms of depression and anxiety.

We will be using some fermented foods in the recipes in this book, but there are numerous options available to help you take advantage of these beneficial foods. Aim for at least one serving of a fermented food each day. Here are some great examples that can be made at home, or you can purchase them at your local grocery store to save time:

- Sauerkraut
- Kimchi
- Kombucha
- Miso
- Tempeh
- Plain yogurt (grass-fed)
- Kefir (grass-fed)
- Fermented pickles
- Apple cider vinegar (with the mother)
- Natto
- Fermented vegetables

FOODS THAT FIGHT INFLAMMATION

Food is a powerful tool when fighting inflammation. Unfortunately, there is no single magic food or nutrient to cure out-of-control inflammation. The beauty of the modified Mediterranean diet for psoriasis is the wide array of delicious anti-inflammatory food choices. Remember, the diet as a whole has the most powerful impact on disease prevention and symptom reversal. Here are some key foods to add to your autoimmune disease–fighting arsenal.

Beans. Beans are high in fiber, which helps feed the gut microbiome. They have antioxidant and anti-inflammatory benefits and are a great plant-based source of protein and minerals. Some people with autoimmune diseases like psoriasis are cautioned to avoid beans because of their lectin content, but when beans are cooked, this is not a concern. Beans can be problematic for some people with an unhealthy gut, but once the gut has healed, beans are a great anti-inflammatory option.

Fruits and vegetables. The Mediterranean diet encourages the consumption of a wide variety of fruits and vegetables. This is a delicious way to improve your intake of dietary fiber, vitamins, minerals, and antioxidants. Fiber improves the health of the gut microbiome and, in turn, helps quiet the inflammatory process. To enjoy the many benefits of a diet rich in fruits and vegetables, variety is key. Aim to include all colors and types. If nightshades are problematic, avoid potatoes, tomatoes, eggplant, and bell peppers.

Gluten-free grains. Whole grains are full of fiber, vitamins, minerals, and phytonutrients and can be a defense against inflammation. They can also assist in blood-sugar regulation. It can be hard to choose true whole grains because, unfortunately, food marketing can be misleading. The recipes in this book will give you some good ideas of the types of grains to choose and how to incorporate them into your daily routine; that said, the psoriasis diet should not be too reliant on grains. Gluten-free grains include amaranth, buckwheat, sorghum, millet, quinoa, buckwheat, teff, brown rice, and oats.

Green tea. The polyphenols in green tea have powerful anti-inflammatory properties. Drink green tea daily and add some ginger or turmeric to enhance the anti-inflammatory effects.

Herbs and spices. Add herbs and spices to your recipes not only for a powerful anti-inflammatory effect, but also to enhance flavor and keep your meal plan exciting. A few of my favorites include turmeric, which has been shown to reduce inflammation; ginger, which is a powerful anti-inflammatory; cinnamon, which has been shown to improve blood glucose and has anti-inflammatory properties; garlic, which can improve arthritis symptoms; and cayenne, which improves circulation and digestion and is an anti-inflammatory (avoid cayenne if you are sensitive to nightshades). Freshly ground black pepper can help quiet inflammation and enhance nutrient absorption. Cloves are a powerful antioxidant and anti-inflammatory, and basil acts as an antioxidant. Coriander can lower blood sugar, and cumin can improve immune system function. Oregano acts as an antioxidant, and rosemary stimulates the immune system and helps digestion. Sage is an anti-inflammatory and antioxidant, and thyme also acts as an antioxidant. Choose a variety of herbs and spices and modify the recipes in this book to create your own unique flavor combinations.

Nuts and seeds. Nuts and seeds are excellent sources of healthy polyunsaturated, monounsaturated, and saturated fats. They are high in fiber, micronutrients, and antioxidants that have a prebiotic effect on the gut microbiome and help reduce chronic inflammation. They also help lower blood sugar and maintain healthy cholesterol levels. Nuts and seeds are filling and make an excellent portable snack. Aim to consume one serving of nuts and seeds each day. Almonds and walnuts are great, but variety is important, so also look for pecans, hazelnuts, Brazil nuts, cashews, pistachios, macadamia nuts, pumpkin seeds, chia seeds, flaxseeds, hemp seeds, and sesame seeds.

Olive oil. The Mediterranean diet is characterized by the liberal use of extra-virgin olive oil. This powerful monounsaturated fat has been researched extensively. According to a 2019 review in *Nutrients*, the benefits are related to its anti-inflammatory, antioxidant, and immune-modulating properties. Extra-virgin olive oil can lower body mass index and blood pressure, as well as help in preventing cancer and reducing the risk of vascular disease. It has also been shown to aid in the treatment of inflammatory autoimmune conditions.

Omega-3 fatty acids. These powerhouse fats counter inflammation by reducing the proteins that trigger an inflammatory response. The two most beneficial forms of omega-3 fatty acids are eicosapentaenoic acid (EPA) and docosahexaenoic acid (DHA), which are found in fatty fish, grass-fed beef, and pasture-raised eggs. Omega-3 fatty acids can't be made by the body, so they must be consumed in the diet. Aim to eat foods high in omega-3 fatty acids such as fatty fish (lake trout, sardines, salmon, etc.) at least twice per week. If you don't like fish, a nutritional supplement may be necessary.

FOODS THAT WORSEN INFLAMMATION

Just as food can be used to reverse the inflammatory process, it can also cause inflammation that leads to diseases like psoriasis. Fortunately, the list of foods that fight inflammation is long and delicious. However, there are a few foods you will likely need to avoid in order to help your body begin to heal.

Dairy. Lactose intolerance is problematic for many people, but those with autoimmune diseases may be more sensitive to dairy products, which can increase inflammation and exacerbate symptoms. If you've never cut dairy out of your diet, try eliminating it for at least two weeks. If you do choose to add it back, look for high-quality grass-fed options. Goat's or sheep's milk is usually better tolerated than regular cow's milk, so those are options if you choose to continue consuming dairy products.

Gluten. Gluten is the protein found in grains such as barley, rye, and wheat. For people with autoimmune diseases, gluten acts like a foreign invader. As the body mounts the defense, it begins to attack its own tissues. People with celiac disease must avoid gluten at all costs, but non-celiac gluten sensitivity increases the inflammatory response and exacerbates the symptoms of numerous diseases. Even people with a healthy gut experience side effects, such as fatigue or bloating, after eating gluten-containing foods.

Soy. Soy can be healthy in a fermented, non–genetically modified form. However, most of the soy products available today are highly processed and create an environment in the body that increases inflammation. Soy in its whole, unprocessed forms (edamame and tofu) and fermented forms (miso and tempeh) can be part of the psoriasis meal plan, but avoid processed forms of soy, such as soybean oil and soy protein isolate.

Nightshades. This subset of vegetables can increase inflammation in some people, especially those with autoimmune disease. Potatoes, tomatoes, eggplant, and bell peppers can cause some people to experience negative symptoms and inflammation. Although these vegetables are packed with nutrients and fiber, you may want to omit them from your diet for a period of time and then reintroduce them in their pure form. Several common spices such as red pepper flakes, cayenne pepper, chili powder, and paprika are also in the nightshade family. Take note of your symptoms—if you experience a flare after consuming any of these foods or spices, then you may need to avoid nightshades.

Processed foods. We live in a convenience culture, but it has been at the expense of our health. Eating real food is the best way to combat this problem. Processed foods that seem healthy may still have some questionable ingredients that will affect the gut microbiome and increase inflammation in the body. We all know to avoid foods with ingredients we can't pronounce, but be sure to check out the ingredient list and, if you see any of the following, think twice before consuming: emulsifiers and gums, such as carrageenan and xanthan gum; hydrogenated and partially hydrogenated oils; corn oil; canola oil; soybean oil; safflower oil; and sunflower oil.

Sugar and artificial sweeteners. We have been told for years that fat is the culprit when it comes to chronic disease, but unfortunately, it's sugar that wreaks the most havoc on the brain and body. Healthy fats are crucial for the body, but sugar is just an indulgence. Sugar, especially processed sugar, is toxic to the gut microbiome, and sugar substitutes are just as damaging. This book contains some recipes with sugar in the form of honey and maple syrup (both of which contain antioxidants, vitamins, and minerals), but for the most part, sugar should be avoided, especially when trying to heal from a chronic disease.

THE PSORIASIS DIET AT A GLANCE

The list of foods to avoid may seem daunting, but once you get the hang of your new way of eating, you'll realize just how many wonderful, delicious anti-inflammatory options you have. You will never get bored with this eating style.

Foods to Enjoy

Fish: anchovies, clams, grouper, halibut, herring, king mackerel, mackerel, marlin, mussels, orange roughy, oysters, salmon, sardines, scallops, sea bass, shark, shrimp, sushi, swordfish, tilefish, tuna, and wild salmon.

Vegetables: virtually any vegetable fits into this meal plan, including arugula, asparagus, beet greens, broccoli, broccoli sprouts, Brussels sprouts, cabbage, carrots, cauliflower, celery, collard greens, cucumbers, dandelion greens, escarole, garlic, kale, kohlrabi, mushrooms, mustard greens, okra, onions, pumpkin, radishes, seaweed, shallots, spinach, sweet potatoes, Swiss chard, turnip greens, watercress, winter squash, and zucchini.

Fruits: açai berries, apples, avocados, bananas, blackberries, blueberries, cherries, coconuts, dragon fruit, goji berries, gooseberries, grapefruits, grapes, kiwifruits, lemons, limes, nectarines, olives, oranges, papaya, peaches, pineapples, plums, pomegranates, raspberries, strawberries, and tangerines.

Beans (if these cause digestive problems, limit or avoid): adzuki beans; baked beans; black beans; black-eyed peas; chickpeas; green beans; kidney beans; lentils; lima beans; mung beans; organic soy-based foods, such as tofu, tempeh, natto, and miso; peas; and snow peas.

Grains: amaranth, black and brown rice, buckwheat, millet, oats (make sure the oats are marked gluten-free to ensure they haven't been cross contaminated during packaging), quinoa, red and wild rice, sorghum, and teff.

Nuts and Seeds: almonds, Brazil nuts, cashews, chia seeds, hazelnuts, hemp seeds, macadamia nuts, pecans, pistachios, plain nut butters, pumpkin seeds, sesame seeds, walnuts, and whole-milled flaxseed.

Fats and Oils: almond oil, avocado oil, coconut oil, extra-virgin olive oil, flax oil, ghee, grass-fed butter, hemp oil, macadamia oil, sesame seed oil, tahini, and walnut oil.

Meat (red meat is very limited on the healing psoriasis diet): small amounts of grass-fed, organic beef, lamb, and venison.

Poultry: organic chicken, turkey, and duck; organic eggs, in small amounts.

Dairy: small amounts of butter or ghee, goat's or sheep's milk, grass-fed whole milk, kefir, unsweetened yogurt, and whole-milk cheeses.

Sugar and Sweeteners: small amounts of coconut sugar, date sugar, erythritol, fresh fruit juice, honey, molasses, monk fruit, organic maple syrup, and stevia.

Beverages: coconut water, coffee, green tea, homemade green smoothies, water, and watermelon water.

Foods to Avoid

Meat: bacon, conventionally raised meat products, deli and processed meats, hot dogs, and sausage.

Poultry: conventionally farmed eggs, conventionally raised poultry, and processed poultry.

Dairy: cheeses made from skim milk or reduced fat milk; conventionally raised dairy; low-fat or nonfat yogurt; processed cheeses; skim, 1%, or 2% milk; and yogurts that contain flavorings and additives.

Fish: farmed fish with antibiotics, hormones, and high levels of toxins. (To find healthy seafood options, go to SeafoodWatch.org.)

Vegetables: if avoiding nightshades, then omit bell peppers; eggplant; white, red, and blue-skinned potatoes; and tomatoes.

Fruit: dried fruit and fruit juice made with sugar.

Beans: GMO soybeans.

Grains: barley, bulgur, couscous, farro, kamut, refined grains, rye, semolina, spelt, and wheat.

Nuts and Seeds: chocolate-covered nuts, nut butters made with unhealthy oils or sugar, and peanuts.

Fats and Oils: canola oil, corn oil, hydrogenated oils, margarine, palm oil, peanut oil, safflower oil, soybean oil, sunflower oil, and vegetable oil.

Sugar and Sweeteners: artificial sweeteners, such as aspartame, sucralose, saccharin, and acesulfame potassium; brown sugar; high-fructose corn syrup; processed foods with added sugars; and white sugar.

Beverages: artificially sweetened coffees, teas, milk, and soda; commercially prepared smoothies and shakes; enhanced waters; and packaged fruit juices.

HOME COOKING MADE EASIER

The best way to work toward better health is to get in the kitchen. Dining out frequently can expose you to trigger foods and inflammatory ingredients and should be avoided. Empower yourself by choosing to cook most of your meals at home to guarantee you'll get the maximum nutrition and have more control over what you're putting into your body. If you've never cooked, there is no need to be intimidated. The psoriasis meal plan provided here is easy to implement and will help you start your healing journey. Once you get the hang of it, you'll actually be excited to experiment in the kitchen. Creating a kitchen that is stocked with basics can be so helpful in keeping you on track. Most of the recipes in this book contain just a few simple ingredients. If your kitchen is well stocked, you'll always have what you need, and cooking will be a breeze.

Must-Haves

Refrigerated and Frozen Items:

- Chicken and turkey (organic and pasture-raised, if available)

- Eggs (cage-free and organic, if available and tolerated)

- Fermented foods: Kefir, kimchi, organic tofu, plain yogurt, sauerkraut, and tempeh

- Fish and seafood (wild-caught, if available): Anchovies, cod, haddock, mussels, oysters, salmon, sardines, shrimp, and tuna

- Fresh fruits and vegetables (organic, if available)

- Frozen fruits and vegetables (organic, if available)

- Grass-fed butter (in small amounts)

- Nut milks: Almond milk, cashew milk, and coconut milk

- Red meat (organic and grass-fed, if available, including limited amounts of ground meat and steak)

Pantry Items:

- Apple cider vinegar (with the mother) and balsamic vinegar

- Coconut cream, coconut milk, and unsweetened coconut flakes

- Coconut sugar, honey, pure maple syrup, and stevia

- Dijon mustard

- Dried or canned beans: Black beans, chickpeas, Great Northern beans, kidney beans, pinto beans

- Flours: Almond flour, cassava flour, gluten-free oat flour, teff flour, and tigernut flour

- Grains: Amaranth, black and brown rice, buckwheat, millet, oats, quinoa, red and wild rice, sorghum, and teff

- Nut butters with no added oils or sugar: Almond butter, cashew butter, and pecan butter

- Nuts: Almonds, Brazil nuts, cashews, hazelnuts, macadamia nuts, pecans, pistachios, and walnuts

- Oils: Avocado, coconut, and extra-virgin olive oils and ghee

- Seeds: Chia seeds, hemp seeds, pumpkin seeds, and whole-milled flaxseed

Herbs and Spices:

- Cayenne pepper, chili powder, and red pepper flakes (if not avoiding nightshades)

- Dried basil, oregano, rosemary, sage, and thyme

- Freshly ground black pepper

- Ground cinnamon, coriander, cloves, cumin, ginger, and turmeric

- Garlic and onion powders

- Kosher salt and sea salt

 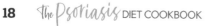

Beverages:

- All varieties of green tea

- Organic coffee

- Sparkling water

Time-Saving Tips

Starting something new, such as cooking your own meals, can be challenging. There's always a learning curve. If you don't feel well or are trying to recover from negative symptoms, adopting these types of lifestyle changes can seem even more daunting. The psoriasis diet is realistic in its approach and the recipes are easy to prepare, but you can also set yourself up for success by learning how to save time in the kitchen. Think about some of the following ideas to help minimize your time in the kitchen while maximizing your results.

Keep an organized work area. If you're like me, the kitchen is a catch-all. Try to keep the kitchen clean and orderly. It is so much more enjoyable to cook in an organized space, and you'll be less likely to get distracted or frustrated when trying new recipes.

Plan your meals for the week and go to the grocery store. It will be so much easier to reach your goals if you're prepared for the week. Set aside some time each week to create a basic menu from the recipes provided, make your grocery list from that menu, and shop from your list once you get to the grocery store. If you have the items on hand to follow through with your menu, you'll have much less stress at mealtime and it will be easier to reach your goals.

Set aside a couple of hours each week to batch cook and do meal prep. Double some of the recipes and portion them out for a few days of lunches or freeze half for another night when time for meal prep is short. You can also wash and pre-cut vegetables for salads and advance cook starches and proteins such as rice, quinoa, and chicken, which can easily be reheated later.

Buy frozen and pre-cut fruits and vegetables. If you're running low on time, make life easier by taking advantage of these shortcuts. For example, instead of buying a head of cauliflower and then going through the process of making riced cauliflower, simply buy frozen cauliflower rice. Many frozen fruits and vegetables contain the same or similar vitamins and nutrients as fresh.

Read recipes completely before starting the cooking process. I have been guilty of just glancing at recipes and then, once I get into it, realizing it's more involved than I expected or that I don't have an ingredient. You'll save yourself so much time if you read the recipe closely before getting started.

ABOUT THE RECIPES

Food is a powerful way to target the root causes of psoriasis. Although it may seem like a daunting task to change your eating habits, it doesn't have to be a stressful process and you can still enjoy delicious foods. Learning how to cook anti-inflammatory meals can be wonderful. Instead of focusing on the foods you may need to avoid, choose instead to be excited about your healing journey and all the flavorful foods that await you.

Even though you will likely have to substitute new foods for some you are used to eating, there is never a need to feel deprived as you embrace your new eating style. The recipes in this book will introduce you to healthy, delicious meals appropriate for the entire family, including Turkey Hash Breakfast Bowls (page 33), Healthy Fish Tacos (page 87), and Walnut-Mushroom Burgers (page 69). Each recipe has been created to help maximize nutrient intake and flavor with affordable, easy-to-find ingredients and step-by-step directions. It can be difficult to spend a lot of time in the kitchen, so the majority of the recipes take 30 minutes or less to prepare, have no more than 10 ingredients, and/or can be prepared in one pot or pan.

There are some additional helpful features that will make menu selections and cooking easier. Each recipe has a label for quick reference. Labels include Gluten-Free, Dairy-Free, Nightshade-Free, Vegetarian, and Vegan. (Even with these labels, you should always read the ingredient label on any packaged food you buy and use in your recipes to ensure all ingredients meet your dietary requirements.) To help you customize your meals, Substitution Tips, Ingredient Tips, Make It Easier Tips, Batch Cook Tips, or Variation Tips are included with many of the recipes. In addition, serving sizes and nutritional information (per serving) are provided.

I am confident you will be able to incorporate these recipes into your new lifestyle and experience symptom improvement along the way. Happy cooking!

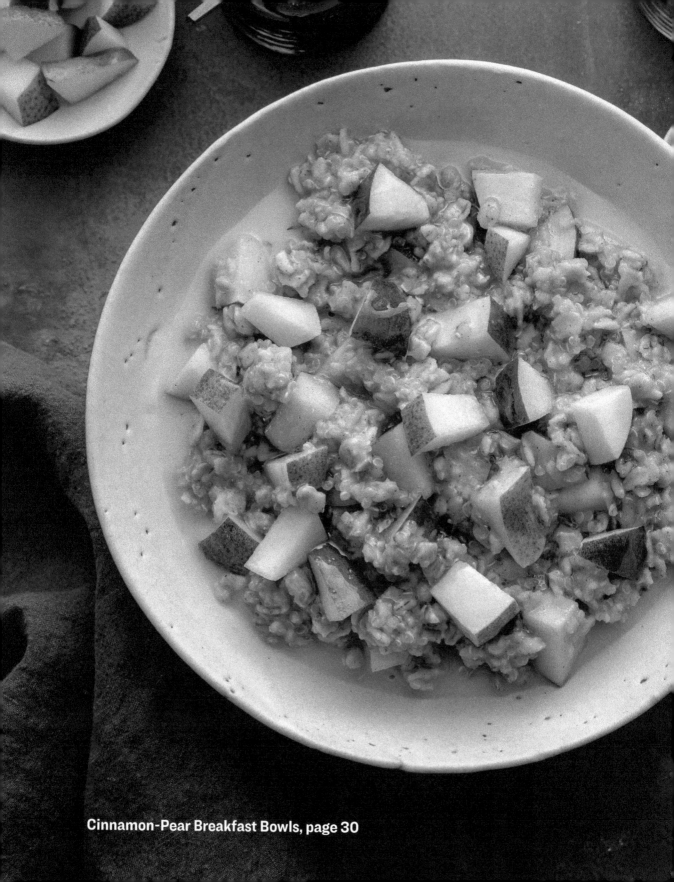

Cinnamon-Pear Breakfast Bowls, page 30

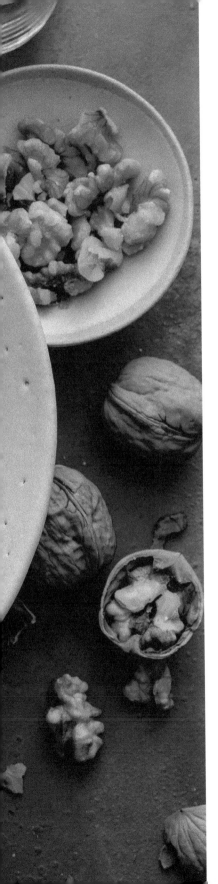

2

SMOOTHIES AND BREAKFASTS

Berry-Plum Smoothie

GLUTEN-FREE • DAIRY-FREE • NIGHTSHADE-FREE • VEGETARIAN

SERVES 2 **PREP** 5 minutes

Green smoothies are a great way to pack nutrients into a portable meal. The options are endless, and it's a super fun opportunity to get creative. This delicious smoothie contains more than a third of your daily fiber requirement, and the blueberries and plum are tangy sources of polyphenols and antioxidants to help fight inflammation. Bonus: The honey adds just a touch of sweetness and helps fight inflammation and boost the immune system.

2½ cups unsweetened vanilla almond milk

2 cups spinach

2 tablespoons chia seeds

2 teaspoons honey

2 teaspoons ground ginger

1 plum, pit removed and frozen in chunks

½ medium avocado, pitted, peeled, and frozen in chunks

1 cup frozen blueberries

1. Put the almond milk, spinach, chia seeds, honey, and ginger into a blender and process for 1 minute.

2. Add the plum, avocado, and blueberries and blend on high for 1 minute.

Make It Easier Tip: I partially prepare my green smoothies the night before: I add all but the frozen ingredients to the blender pitcher and let it sit in the refrigerator overnight. In the morning, I just add the frozen ingredients, blend it up, and go!

Per serving (10 ounces): Calories: 282, Total Fat: 15g, Saturated Fat: 1g, Cholesterol: 0mg, Sodium: 256mg, Carbohydrates: 35g, Fiber: 12g, Protein: 6g

Pumpkin Pie Smoothie

GLUTEN-FREE • DAIRY-FREE • NIGHTSHADE-FREE • VEGETARIAN

SERVES 2 **PREP** 5 minutes

We normally save pumpkin for our favorite fall dishes, but you can enjoy it all year long in this nutrient-packed, mouthwatering, anti-inflammatory smoothie. Pumpkins are a great source of fiber in a low-calorie package and contain valuable vitamins and minerals.

2½ cups unsweetened vanilla almond milk

2 cups spinach

2 tablespoons whole-milled flaxseed

2 teaspoons honey

1 teaspoon ground cinnamon

1 teaspoon ground cloves

1 teaspoon ground nutmeg

1 teaspoon vanilla extract

1 small banana, frozen

½ cup canned pumpkin, frozen

1. Put the almond milk, spinach, flaxseed, honey, cinnamon, cloves, nutmeg, and vanilla into a blender and process for 1 minute.

2. Add the banana and pumpkin and blend on high for 1 minute.

Variation Tip: Add ½ medium avocado, pitted, peeled, and frozen in chunks, to increase the fiber and healthy fat in this smoothie.

Per serving (10 ounces): Calories: 236, Total Fat: 11g, Saturated Fat: 2g, Cholesterol: 0mg, Sodium: 270mg, Carbohydrates: 32g, Fiber: 10g, Protein: 7g

Nutty Chocolate Smoothie

GLUTEN-FREE • DAIRY-FREE • NIGHTSHADE-FREE • VEGETARIAN

SERVES 2   **PREP** 5 minutes

Milkshakes taste great but are often made with inflammatory ingredients. With this smoothie, you can enjoy the flavor of a chocolate milkshake and promote good health at the same time. Nut butters provide anti-inflammatory fats, and the cacao powder and blueberries are great sources of anti-inflammatory flavonoids. Look for nut butters with no added sugar or oils. I like to use pecan butter, but almond or cashew butter work well, too. As a bonus, this smoothie provides about half the fiber you need each day to maintain a healthy gut microbiome.

2½ cups unsweetened vanilla almond milk

2 cups spinach

6 baby carrots

2 tablespoons nut butter

2 tablespoons cacao powder

2 tablespoons chia seeds

2 teaspoons honey

1 teaspoon vanilla extract

½ medium avocado, pitted, peeled, and frozen in chunks

½ frozen banana

½ cup frozen blueberries

1. Put the almond milk, spinach, carrots, nut butter, cacao powder, chia seeds, honey, and vanilla into a blender and process for 1 minute.

2. Add the avocado, banana, and blueberries to the blender and blend on high for 1 minute.

Ingredient Tip: Cocoa is the processed form of cacao. Although both contain antioxidants, vitamins, and minerals, the less-processed cacao provides a more powerful nutritional punch. If you choose cocoa, look for the unsweetened variety.

Per serving (10 ounces): Calories: 427, Total Fat: 27g, Saturated Fat: 6g, Cholesterol: 0mg, Sodium: 281mg, Carbohydrates: 48g, Fiber: 19g, Protein: 13g

Cinnamon-Nectarine Smoothie

GLUTEN-FREE • DAIRY-FREE • NIGHTSHADE-FREE • VEGETARIAN

SERVES 2   **PREP** 5 minutes

This smoothie is filled with anti-inflammatory nutrients but tastes so good it will have you wondering if it's actually psoriasis-diet legal! The nectarine, avocado, and whole-milled flaxseed contain fiber to help feed your good gut bacteria and control your blood sugar. The combination of ginger, cinnamon, and honey is both delicious and inflammation fighting.

2½ cups unsweetened vanilla almond milk

2 cups spinach

1 celery stalk, cut in half horizontally

2 tablespoons freshly squeezed lemon juice

2 tablespoons whole-milled flaxseed

2 teaspoons honey

½ teaspoon ground cinnamon

½ teaspoon ground ginger

1 nectarine, pit removed and frozen in chunks

½ medium avocado, pitted, peeled, and frozen in chunks

1. Put the almond milk, spinach, celery, lemon juice, flaxseed, honey, cinnamon, and ginger into a blender and process for 1 minute.

2. Add the nectarine and avocado and blend on high for 1 minute.

Variation Tip: Use kale or collard greens (with their stems removed) in place of the spinach for an extra boost of dark, leafy greens.

Per serving (10 ounces): Calories: 228, Total Fat: 14g, Saturated Fat: 1g, Cholesterol: 0mg, Sodium: 272mg, Carbohydrates: 24g, Fiber: 9g, Protein: 5g

Strawberry "Milkshake" Smoothie

GLUTEN-FREE • DAIRY-FREE • NIGHTSHADE-FREE • VEGETARIAN

SERVES 2   **PREP** 5 minutes

I created this creamy smoothie for my husband because he loves all things strawberry. It's simple to whip up and can be enjoyed for breakfast or as an after-dinner treat. Chia seeds are loaded with fiber, healthy fat, and protein and have been shown to help reduce inflammation and help control blood sugar.

2½ cups unsweetened vanilla almond milk

2 cups spinach

1 celery stalk

2 tablespoons chia seeds

2 teaspoons honey

6 medium frozen strawberries

½ medium banana, frozen

1. Put the almond milk, spinach, celery, chia seeds, and honey into a blender and process for 1 minute.

2. Add the strawberries and the banana and blend on high for 1 minute.

Ingredient Tip: Instead of ice, I use frozen fruit in my green smoothies. Pre-packaged frozen fruit is convenient, but I often freeze my own fruit, which saves a little money and helps prevent food waste. For bananas, I peel and break them in half before freezing. For avocados and stone fruit, I wash them, cut them in half, remove the pit, and chop them into chunks.

Per serving (10 ounces): Calories: 188, Total Fat: 8g, Saturated Fat: 1g, Cholesterol: 0mg, Sodium: 268mg, Carbohydrates: 26g, Fiber: 9g, Protein: 5g

Apple-Coconut Quinoa

GLUTEN-FREE • DAIRY-FREE • NIGHTSHADE-FREE • VEGAN

SERVES 4 **PREP** 5 minutes **COOK** 15 minutes

Oats aren't the only filling grain option for breakfast. Quinoa (actually a seed) is usually served as part of, or alongside, a lunch or dinner dish, but this recipe will have you thinking of it as your new favorite breakfast food. This slightly sweet, hearty dish can be served hot or cold and is a good source of fiber and B vitamins. It is also packed with plant-based protein to keep you alert for the day ahead.

1 cup quinoa, rinsed and drained

2½ cups unsweetened vanilla almond milk

⅛ teaspoon kosher salt

2 tablespoons pure maple syrup

1 Gala apple, chopped, for topping

¼ cup unsweetened shredded coconut, for topping

¼ cup chopped walnuts, for topping

1. In a large saucepan, combine the quinoa, almond milk, and salt. Mix well.

2. Bring the quinoa mixture to a boil over medium heat. Cover, reduce the heat to low, and simmer for 12 minutes.

3. Remove the lid from the pot, stir the quinoa, and cook, uncovered, for 3 more minutes.

4. Remove the quinoa mixture from the heat and stir in the maple syrup.

5. Divide the quinoa mixture among 4 bowls and top with the apple, coconut, and walnuts.

Ingredient Tip: Quinoa needs to be rinsed well prior to cooking to remove the saponin, an outer coating that can have a bitter or soapy taste. Using a fine-mesh strainer is the easiest method.

Per serving (¾ cup): Calories: 326, Total Fat: 14g, Saturated Fat: 4g, Cholesterol: 0mg, Sodium: 177mg, Carbohydrates: 43g, Fiber: 6g, Protein: 8g

Cinnamon-Pear Breakfast Bowls

GLUTEN-FREE • DAIRY-FREE • NIGHTSHADE-FREE • VEGETARIAN

SERVES 2   **PREP** 5 minutes   **COOK** 5 minutes

On hectic mornings, breakfast can easily be forgotten. This slightly sweet and savory option will keep the meal front and center. This nutritious dish has a good amount of protein and is high in fiber to help you feel full all morning.

¾ cup gluten-free rolled oats

2 cups unsweetened vanilla almond milk

½ cup cooked quinoa

1 pear, thinly sliced

2 tablespoons chopped walnuts

¼ teaspoon ground cinnamon

Honey or maple syrup, for topping

1. In a medium microwave-safe bowl, combine the oats and almond milk and mix well.

2. Microwave, uncovered, for 1 to 2 minutes, or until the oatmeal thickens.

3. Remove the oatmeal from the microwave and mix in the cooked quinoa, sliced pear, walnuts, and cinnamon.

4. Divide the mixture between 2 bowls.

5. Drizzle honey or maple syrup over top of each serving.

Make It Easier Tip: Prepare a large batch of quinoa ahead of time and store for up to 5 days in the refrigerator so you can use it in a variety of anti-inflammatory recipes all week long.

Per serving (½ cup): Calories: 419, Total Fat: 13g, Saturated Fat: 1g,

Cholesterol: 0mg, Sodium: 96mg, Carbohydrates: 65g, Fiber: 11g, Protein: 13g

Easy Overnight Oats

GLUTEN-FREE • DAIRY-FREE • NIGHTSHADE-FREE • VEGAN

SERVES 2   **PREP** 10 minutes, plus overnight to soak

Oatmeal is the quintessential breakfast food, but it doesn't have to be boring. This is another versatile, scrumptious recipe that can be changed depending on your mood. I like to mix and match the fruit, nut, and seed combinations in this dish and sometimes even add in a few small chunks of dark chocolate. Packed with nutrients and fiber, these oats are also super convenient and travel well.

1 cup gluten-free rolled oats

½ cup unsweetened vanilla almond milk

1 tablespoon maple syrup, plus more for topping

2 teaspoons chia seeds, plus more for topping

½ teaspoon ground cinnamon

1 Gala apple, cored and diced, for topping

¼ cup chopped pecans, for topping

1. In a large bowl, combine the oats, almond milk, maple syrup, chia seeds, and cinnamon. Mix well, then cover and let the oats soak in the refrigerator overnight.

2. In the morning, divide the oatmeal between 2 bowls and top with equal amounts of the apple and pecans.

3. Sprinkle with additional chia seeds and a drizzle of maple syrup before serving.

Batch Cook Tip: Triple the recipe and make enough overnight oats for several breakfasts. When you are preparing the oats, simply portion them out into separate individual containers (I use mason jars) so you can grab one on your way out the door.

Per serving (½ cup): Calories: 365, Total Fat: 16g, Saturated Fat: 2g, Cholesterol: 0mg, Sodium: 47mg, Carbohydrates: 53g, Fiber: 11g, Protein: 8g

Zucchini-Pepper Egg Muffins

GLUTEN-FREE • DAIRY-FREE • VEGETARIAN

SERVES 4   **PREP** 10 minutes   **COOK** 30 minutes

If eggs are included in your meal plan, try these delightful egg muffins. They're a great way to increase your intake of healthy anti-inflammatory fats and vegetables, and they are also a perfect source of protein to help keep you feeling full until lunchtime. This recipe is simple and portable for hectic mornings.

Coconut oil, melted, for greasing the tin

12 large eggs

¼ teaspoon dried oregano

¼ teaspoon dried basil

¼ teaspoon dried thyme

¼ teaspoon kosher salt

¼ teaspoon freshly ground black pepper

½ large zucchini, diced

6 small bell peppers, diced

1 small onion, diced

1. Preheat the oven to 350°F and grease a muffin tin with melted coconut oil.

2. Crack the eggs into a large bowl, then add the oregano, basil, thyme, salt, and black pepper and whisk until well combined.

3. Add the zucchini, bell peppers, and onion to the egg mixture and mix well.

4. Pour ¼ cup of the egg mixture into each of the 12 muffin cups. (If you have extra, divide it evenly among the muffin cups.)

5. Bake for 30 minutes.

6. Remove from the oven and allow to cool slightly before serving or storing.

Substitution Tip: If avoiding nightshades, omit the bell peppers and add another favorite vegetable. Chopped broccoli florets would be a perfect addition here.

Per serving (3 egg muffins): Calories: 225, Total Fat: 13g, Saturated Fat: 4g, Cholesterol: 491mg, Sodium: 310mg, Carbohydrates: 9g, Fiber: 3g, Protein: 18g

Turkey Hash Breakfast Bowls

GLUTEN-FREE • DAIRY-FREE

SERVES 4 **PREP** 5 minutes **COOK** 20 minutes

Forget about turkey bacon and check out these yummy anti-inflammatory turkey bowls! You can savor the combination of herbs, spices, and vegetables for breakfast, but this dish is also a great lunch or dinner meal.

2 tablespoons avocado oil, divided

1 yellow onion, diced

2 garlic cloves, chopped

1 pound ground turkey

½ teaspoon dried thyme

¼ teaspoon dried oregano

½ teaspoon freshly ground black pepper

1 teaspoon ground turmeric

¼ teaspoon kosher salt

1 zucchini, diced

1 yellow squash, diced

1 red bell pepper, diced

1. In a large skillet over high heat, warm 1 tablespoon of the avocado oil.

2. Add the onion and garlic and sauté for about 4 minutes.

3. Add the ground turkey, then sprinkle the thyme, oregano, black pepper, turmeric, and salt over the turkey and mix well to combine. Cook until the turkey is done, about 7 minutes.

4. Meanwhile, in another skillet, add the remaining 1 tablespoon avocado oil and sauté the zucchini, yellow squash, and bell pepper for about 7 minutes, or until the vegetables have softened.

5. In a large bowl, combine the turkey with the vegetable mixture.

6. Divide the hash evenly among 4 bowls and serve.

Substitution Tip: If avoiding nightshades, omit the bell pepper and add another favorite vegetable. Diced carrots or chopped mushrooms are great options.

Per serving (1½ cups): Calories: 332, Total Fat: 24g, Saturated Fat: 7g, Cholesterol: 100mg, Sodium: 235mg, Carbohydrates: 9g, Fiber: 2g, Protein: 20g

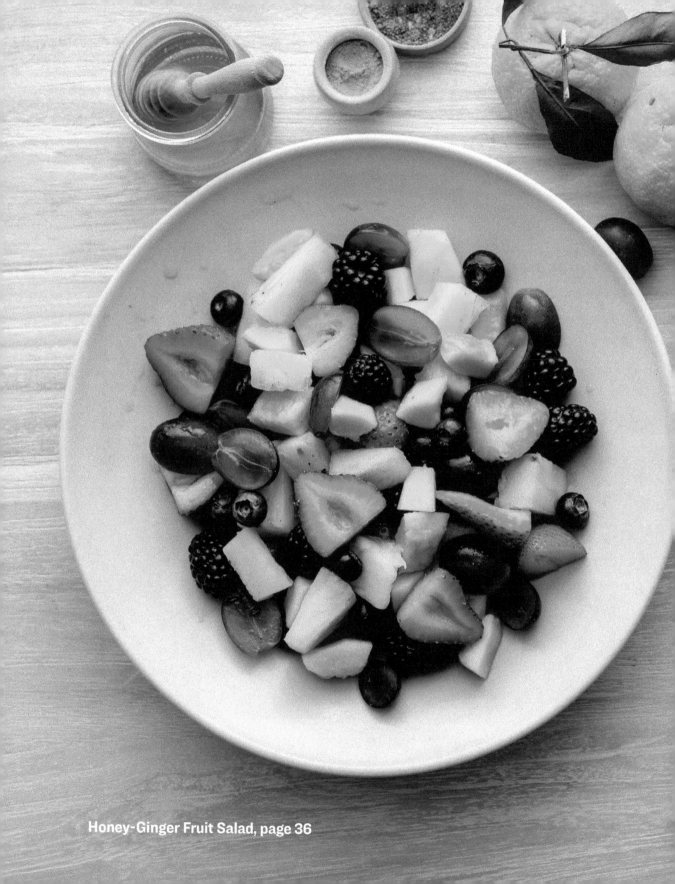

Honey-Ginger Fruit Salad, page 36

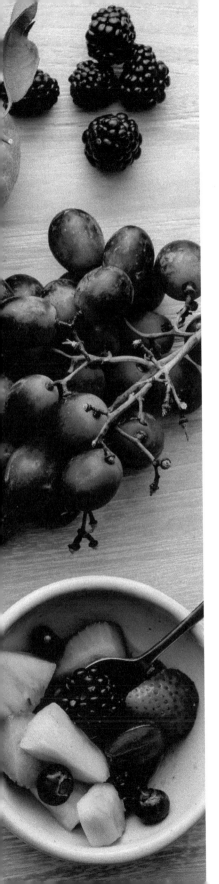

3

SNACKS AND SIDES

Honey-Ginger Fruit Salad

GLUTEN-FREE • DAIRY-FREE • NIGHTSHADE-FREE • VEGETARIAN

SERVES 3   **PREP** 10 minutes, plus 1 hour to chill

If you're looking for a refreshing, light snack or dessert, this recipe has you covered. The power of vitamin C in the fruit and the anti-inflammatory and immune-boosting properties of the ginger and honey create the ideal satisfyingly sweet treat!

¼ cup pineapple chunks

¼ cup blackberries

¼ cup blueberries

¼ cup papaya chunks

5 strawberries, halved

¼ cup grapes

1 tablespoon honey

½ cup freshly squeezed orange juice

1 teaspoon ground ginger

⅛ teaspoon nutmeg

2 tablespoons lemon juice

1. In a large bowl, combine the pineapple, blackberries, blueberries, papaya, strawberries, and grapes.

2. In a small bowl, whisk together the honey, orange juice, ginger, nutmeg, and lemon juice.

3. Pour the dressing over the fruit and toss gently.

4. Cover and chill for 1 hour prior to serving.

> **Variation Tip:** Serve with chopped pecans or walnuts for a more filling snack.

Per serving (¾ cup): Calories: 80, Total Fat: 0g, Saturated Fat: 0g, Cholesterol: 0mg, Sodium: 7mg, Carbohydrates: 20g, Fiber: 2g, Protein: 1g

Black Bean Hummus

GLUTEN-FREE • DAIRY-FREE • NIGHTSHADE-FREE • VEGAN

MAKES 3½ cups   **PREP** 10 minutes

I love experimenting with traditional recipes. Instead of using only chickpeas, I add black beans to take this hummus to the next level. This mouthwatering hummus provides an awesome amount of fiber while also taking advantage of all the wonderful anti-inflammatory benefits of extra-virgin olive oil. Try it for your next snack session.

1 (15-ounce) can chickpeas, half the liquid reserved, then rinsed and drained

1 (15-ounce) can black beans, rinsed and drained

3 garlic cloves

¼ cup extra-virgin olive oil

¼ teaspoon kosher salt

½ teaspoon freshly ground black pepper

1. Put the chickpeas, reserved chickpea water, black beans, garlic, olive oil, salt, and pepper into a food processor or blender and mix on high until smooth.

2. Store in an airtight container in the refrigerator for up to 5 days.

Ingredient Tip: Aquafaba, the liquid from a can of chickpeas (or white beans), can be used as an egg substitute in many recipes. Instead of discarding the liquid from your canned chickpeas, reserve it and freeze it in ice cube trays for later use. When you come across a recipe it would be useful in, simply remove it from the freezer and allow to thaw. Substitute 3 tablespoons aquafaba for 1 whole large egg.

Per serving (¼ cup): Calories: 85, Total Fat: 4g, Saturated Fat: 1g,

Cholesterol: 0mg, Sodium: 37mg, Carbohydrates: 10g, Fiber: 3g, Protein: 3g

Simple Trail Mix

GLUTEN-FREE • NIGHTSHADE-FREE • VEGETARIAN

SERVES 8   **PREP** 10 minutes

You've probably heard that nuts and seeds have too many calories, but never fear! Nuts and seeds are fabulous sources of healthy fats and are loaded with powerful antioxidants, magnesium, and selenium. They can also help reduce inflammatory markers. The possibilities with this trail mix are endless—you can mix and match any nuts and seeds to create different flavors each time. I usually make a batch over the weekend and portion it into quarter-cup packets for a healthy, filling work snack to enjoy throughout the week.

¼ cup cashews

¼ cup pumpkin seeds

¼ cup pecans

¼ cup almonds

¼ cup macadamia nuts

¼ cup walnuts

¼ cup dark chocolate chips (>70% dark chocolate)

¼ cup dried cranberries

1. In a large bowl, combine the cashews, pumpkin seeds, pecans, almonds, macadamia nuts, walnuts, chocolate chips, and cranberries.

2. Portion out into quarter-cup containers.

3. Store in an airtight container in the refrigerator for up to 1 month.

Ingredient Tip: Choose raw nuts or nuts dry roasted without added inflammatory oils.

Per serving (¼ cup): Calories: 170, Total Fat: 14g, Saturated Fat: 2g,

Cholesterol: 0mg, Sodium: 2mg, Carbohydrates: 10g, Fiber: 2g, Protein: 4g

Crispy Kale Chips

GLUTEN-FREE • DAIRY-FREE • NIGHTSHADE-FREE • VEGAN

SERVES 4   **PREP** 5 minutes   **COOK** 25 minutes

Confession time: I love potato chips! There's something about the crunchy texture and salty flavor that calls to me. Unfortunately, store-bought chips typically contain inflammatory oils and other questionable ingredients. This recipe lets you enjoy the best of both worlds: the anti-inflammatory nutrition of kale in the form of a delicious, crunchy chip.

4 cups kale, stemmed and torn into medium-size pieces

2 tablespoons coconut oil, melted

¼ teaspoon kosher salt

1 teaspoon ground cumin

1 teaspoon ground turmeric

1. Preheat the oven to 225°F. Line a baking sheet with parchment paper.

2. Make sure the kale pieces are thoroughly dry, then place the kale in a large bowl.

3. Drizzle with the coconut oil and sprinkle the salt, cumin, and turmeric over the kale. Using clean hands, massage the oil and spices into the kale until the leaves are completely coated.

4. Place the kale on the baking sheet in a single layer. (You may need two lined baking sheets to keep the pieces in one layer.)

5. Bake for 15 minutes, then stir the kale and bake for another 5 to 10 minutes, or until crispy.

6. Remove from the oven and let cool for about 5 minutes.

7. These chips are best when served immediately.

Variation Tip: Choose your favorite spice combination to create your own unique kale chip flavor.

Per serving (2 cups): Calories: 96, Total Fat: 7g, Saturated Fat: 6g, Cholesterol: 0mg, Sodium: 147mg, Carbohydrates: 8g, Fiber: 1g, Protein: 2g

Simple Turmeric Roasted Carrots

GLUTEN-FREE • DAIRY-FREE • NIGHTSHADE-FREE • VEGAN

SERVES 4   **PREP** 5 minutes   **COOK** 25 minutes

Carrots are a versatile root vegetable that contain vitamin A in the form of beta-carotene, as well as fiber. These roasted carrots are the perfect side dish, as they pack a hefty nutritional punch. Turmeric contains curcumin, which is a powerful anti-inflammatory and antioxidant, and the black pepper aids the body's ability to absorb curcumin.

4 large carrots

2 tablespoons extra-virgin olive oil

½ tablespoon ground turmeric

1 teaspoon kosher salt

½ tablespoon freshly ground black pepper

1. Preheat the oven to 400°F. Line a baking sheet with parchment paper.

2. Slice the carrots lengthwise and place them on the baking sheet.

3. In a small bowl, mix together the olive oil, turmeric, salt, and pepper.

4. Using a pastry brush, coat both sides of the carrots with the seasoned olive oil.

5. Bake for 25 minutes, or until the carrots have reached your desired tenderness.

Batch Cook Tip: Double the recipe and freeze the extras for a quick side dish when life gets hectic. To reheat from frozen, simply add the carrots to a saucepan over low heat. You can also chop any leftover carrots and add them to a batch of soup.

Per serving (1 cup): Calories: 95, Total Fat: 7g, Saturated Fat: 1g, Cholesterol: 0mg, Sodium: 518mg, Carbohydrates: 8g, Fiber: 2g, Protein: 1g

Creamy Cauliflower Mash

GLUTEN-FREE • DAIRY-FREE • NIGHTSHADE-FREE • VEGAN

SERVES 4   **PREP** 10 minutes   **COOK** 10 minutes

My mom's mashed potatoes are what dreams are made of, but if you need to avoid dairy and nightshades, traditional mashed potatoes are out. Thankfully, you can enjoy this creamy side dish that tastes great and delivers powerful anti-inflammatory nutrition. Cauliflower contains several antioxidants that can help reduce inflammation and is a great low-carbohydrate grain substitute.

1 medium head cauliflower

2 tablespoons extra-virgin olive oil

1 teaspoon minced fresh garlic

¼ cup full-fat coconut milk

1 teaspoon kosher salt

¼ teaspoon freshly ground black pepper

1. Roughly chop the cauliflower into bite-size florets.

2. In a medium saucepan, bring 1 cup water to a simmer over medium heat. Place the florets in a steamer basket set into the saucepan. Cover the pot and let the cauliflower steam for 8 minutes, or until very soft. Drain well.

3. Put the drained cauliflower chunks into a food processor.

4. Add the olive oil, garlic, coconut milk, salt, and pepper and process until smooth. Serve immediately.

Make It Easier Tip: Instead of fresh cauliflower, you can use frozen riced cauliflower. Simply prepare the riced cauliflower according to the package directions, then add it and the remaining ingredients to your food processer and blend until smooth.

Per serving (¾ cup): Calories: 125, Total Fat: 10g, Saturated Fat: 4g, Cholesterol: 0mg, Sodium: 513mg, Carbohydrates: 8g, Fiber: 4g, Protein: 3g

Wilted Swiss Chard with Red Onion and Garlic

GLUTEN-FREE • DAIRY-FREE • NIGHTSHADE-FREE • VEGAN

SERVES 4   **PREP** 10 minutes   **COOK** 15 minutes

Greens, greens, and more greens! Greens are loaded with powerful antioxidants and fiber to help reduce inflammation and feed the gut microbiome. Swiss chard can be found in the produce section at the grocery store and is either entirely green or green with a red stalk. Here, it makes a fantastic side dish (and the leaves are also great in smoothies).

2 tablespoons avocado oil

1 medium red onion, chopped

2 garlic cloves, chopped

¼ cup apple cider vinegar (with the mother)

4 cups chopped Swiss chard

1 teaspoon kosher salt

¼ teaspoon freshly ground black pepper

1. In a medium saucepan or stockpot over medium heat, combine the avocado oil, onion, garlic, and vinegar.

2. Sauté until the onion is soft and the garlic is fragrant, about 3 minutes.

3. Add one-quarter of the Swiss chard to the pan. When the greens are wilted, repeat this process, until all the greens have been incorporated.

4. Add 1 cup water, cover, and cook for about 10 minutes, stirring halfway through.

5. Season with salt and pepper and serve immediately.

Ingredient Tip: Apple cider vinegar is a fermented food option that can help support gut health. Look for raw, unfiltered varieties "with the mother," indicating the presence of beneficial probiotic bacteria.

Per serving (1 cup): Calories: 86, Total Fat: 7g, Saturated Fat: 1g, Cholesterol: 0mg, Sodium: 547mg, Carbohydrates: 5g, Fiber: 1g, Protein: 1g

Spaghetti Squash with Broccoli

GLUTEN-FREE • DAIRY-FREE • NIGHTSHADE-FREE • VEGAN

SERVES 2   **PREP** 5 minutes   **COOK** 55 minutes

Spaghetti squash is another nutritious vegetable that can be used as a grain alternative. For this recipe, I also like to use broccoli, which contains bioactive compounds to reduce inflammation and is a great source of antioxidants, vitamins, minerals, and fiber. Serve this as a side dish or an entrée.

1 small spaghetti squash, halved lengthwise and seeded

1 tablespoon extra-virgin olive oil

1 head broccoli, cut into bite-size florets

2 tablespoons freshly squeezed lemon juice

2 garlic cloves, chopped

1 teaspoon thyme

½ teaspoon kosher salt

¼ teaspoon freshly ground black pepper

3 tablespoons slivered almonds, for topping

1. Preheat the oven to 375°F. Line a baking sheet with parchment paper.

2. Using a pastry brush, coat the cut side of each squash half with olive oil.

3. Place the squash, cut-sides down, on the baking sheet and roast for 35 minutes, or until fork-tender.

4. Meanwhile, steam the broccoli for 7 minutes, or until firm-tender and bright green.

5. In a small bowl, whisk together the lemon juice, garlic, thyme, salt, and pepper.

6. Remove the squash from the oven and use a fork to scrape the flesh into long, spaghetti-like tendrils.

7. Add half of the broccoli to each squash half, then drizzle each with half of the lemon dressing. Return the squash halves to the oven and bake for 10 minutes.

8. To serve, top each half with slivered almonds.

Ingredient Tip: You can make spaghetti squash ahead of time and store it in the refrigerator. You can also microwave it to save time. Pierce the squash several times, microwave for 10 minutes, rotate, and microwave again for 10 more minutes. Slice in half after cooking and proceed with the recipe, starting at step 4.

Per serving (1½ cups): Calories: 259, Total Fat: 15g, Saturated Fat: 2g, Cholesterol: 0mg, Sodium: 564mg, Carbohydrates: 31g, Fiber: 5g, Protein: 9g

Savory Roasted Herbed Vegetables

GLUTEN-FREE • DAIRY-FREE • NIGHTSHADE-FREE • VEGAN

SERVES 4   **PREP** 10 minutes   **COOK** 30 minutes

This is the ideal wholesome addition to any meal. The cinnamon, nutmeg, and rosemary bring depth and a hint of nutty sweetness to the nutritious root vegetables and Brussels sprouts.

2 medium sweet potatoes, halved and cut into 1-inch cubes

4 medium carrots, cut lengthwise and then into 1-inch chunks

1 pound Brussels sprouts, trimmed and halved

2 tablespoons avocado oil

⅛ teaspoon ground cinnamon

⅛ teaspoon ground nutmeg

¼ teaspoon dried rosemary

¼ teaspoon kosher salt

¼ teaspoon freshly ground black pepper

1. Preheat the oven to 425°F. Line a baking sheet with parchment paper.

2. In a large bowl, combine the sweet potatoes, carrots, and Brussels sprouts.

3. In a small bowl, whisk together the avocado oil, cinnamon, nutmeg, rosemary, salt, and pepper.

4. Pour the dressing over the vegetables and toss well to combine.

5. Spread the vegetables on the baking sheet in a single layer.

6. Bake for 30 minutes, turning every 10 minutes, until vegetables are tender and lightly browned.

Variation Tip: Add chopped onion or cubed parsnips for a different flavor profile.

Per serving (1½ cups): Calories: 191, Total Fat: 8g, Saturated Fat: 1g, Cholesterol: 0mg, Sodium: 223mg, Carbohydrates: 30g, Fiber: 8g, Protein: 5g

Chunky Kohlrabi Slaw

GLUTEN-FREE • DAIRY-FREE • NIGHTSHADE-FREE • VEGAN

SERVES 4 **PREP** 10 minutes

This tangy recipe is the perfect side dish, but sometimes I just eat it as a healthy, refreshing snack! If you've never tried kohlrabi, you're in for a treat. It's a cruciferous (I love that word) vegetable, so it is a powerful source of phytonutrients that are important for lowering inflammation. It can be eaten cooked or raw, and the leaves can be cooked like any other leafy green or added to green smoothies. I like a green apple for this recipe, but feel free to use your favorite variety.

2 small kohlrabi, peeled and shredded

1 large apple, cored and shredded

3 tablespoons chopped pecans

2 tablespoons freshly squeezed lemon juice

2 tablespoons extra-virgin olive oil

2 tablespoons apple cider vinegar (with the mother)

¼ teaspoon kosher salt

¼ teaspoon freshly ground black pepper

In a large bowl, combine the kohlrabi, apple, pecans, lemon juice, olive oil, vinegar, salt, and pepper and mix well. Serve immediately.

Ingredient Tip: Kohlrabi is found near the other greens in the grocery store. You'll need to shave or peel the outer layer of the kohlrabi prior to use.

Per serving (½ cup): Calories: 169, Total Fat: 11g, Saturated Fat: 2g,

Cholesterol: 0mg, Sodium: 146mg, Carbohydrates: 17g, Fiber: 7g, Protein: 3g

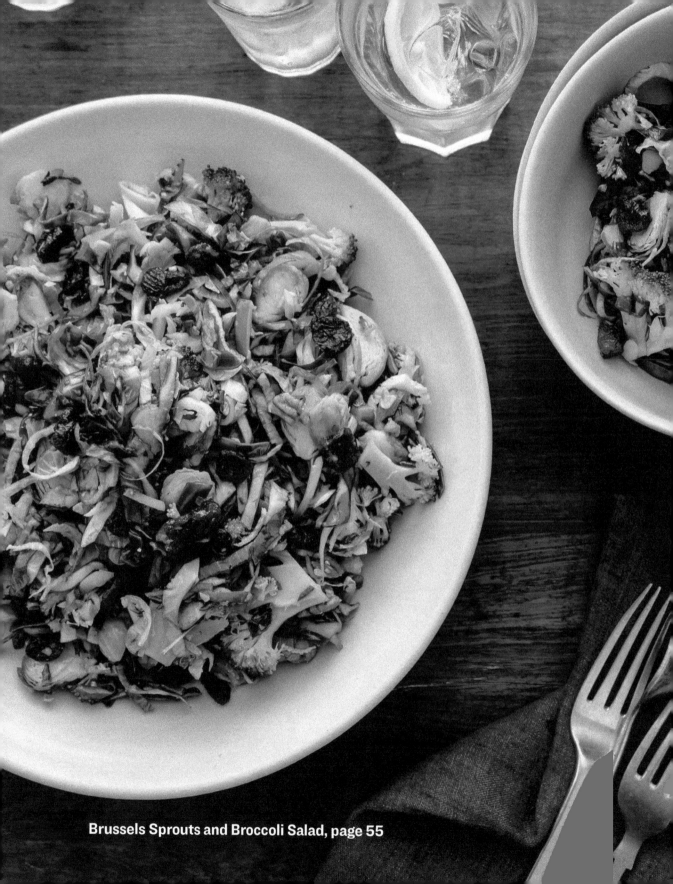

Brussels Sprouts and Broccoli Salad, page 55

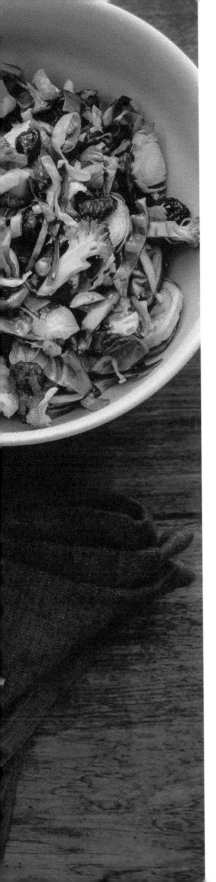

4

SOUPS AND SALADS

Tomato-Free Bean and Veggie Soup

GLUTEN-FREE • DAIRY-FREE • NIGHTSHADE-FREE • VEGAN

SERVES 6   **PREP** 10 minutes   **COOK** 25 minutes

There's nothing better than a warm bowl of homemade vegetable soup, and this chunky tomato-free version is no exception! Soups are a great way to pack in nutrients in a portable, convenient package year-round. Hint: Eat soup for breakfast to get a jump-start on your vegetable servings for the day!

1 tablespoon coconut oil

2 small onions, chopped

3 garlic cloves, chopped

4 cups low-sodium vegetable broth

¼ small red cabbage, shredded

1 medium zucchini, diced

2 cups carrots, diced

½ teaspoon celery salt

1 teaspoon ground cumin

¼ teaspoon kosher salt

½ teaspoon freshly ground black pepper

2 (15-ounce) cans Great Northern beans, rinsed and drained

1. In a large stockpot or Dutch oven over medium-high heat, warm the coconut oil.

2. Add the onions and garlic and sauté until fragrant, about 3 minutes.

3. Add the broth, cabbage, zucchini, carrots, celery salt, cumin, salt, pepper, and 2 cups water.

4. Bring to a boil, then cover and reduce the heat to low. Let the soup simmer for 10 minutes.

5. Add the beans and simmer on low for 10 more minutes, then serve.

Batch Cook Tip: This recipe freezes well, so double the amount and freeze the extras for hectic days when you just don't have time to cook dinner. You can also freeze individual containers for an easy grab-and-go prepped lunch.

Per serving (1 cup): Calories: 175, Total Fat: 3g, Saturated Fat: 2g, Cholesterol: 0mg, Sodium: 160mg, Carbohydrates: 29g, Fiber: 9g, Protein: 10g

Savory Lentil Soup

GLUTEN-FREE • DAIRY-FREE • NIGHTSHADE-FREE • VEGAN

SERVES 6 **PREP** 10 minutes **COOK** 30 minutes

Lentils are little plant-based nutrient dynamos that can be added to a variety of recipes, including soups, stews, salads, burgers, and (believe it or not) desserts. In addition to their high fiber and protein content, lentils also provide B vitamins, iron, and magnesium and are extremely budget-friendly!

¼ cup extra-virgin olive oil

1 yellow onion, chopped

2 carrots, diced

2 celery stalks, chopped

2 garlic cloves, minced

1 teaspoon dried oregano

1 teaspoon dried basil

2 (15-ounce) cans of lentils, rinsed and drained

4 cups low-sodium vegetable broth

1½ cups thinly chopped kale

Kosher salt (optional)

Freshly ground black pepper (optional)

1. In a large stockpot over medium heat, warm the olive oil.

2. Add the onion, carrots, and celery and cook until tender, about 5 minutes.

3. Add the garlic, oregano, and basil and cook for 2 minutes.

4. Add the lentils and broth and bring the mixture to a boil.

5. Reduce the heat to low and simmer for 15 minutes.

6. Just before serving, stir in the kale and cook until it wilts, about 3 minutes.

7. Season with salt and pepper, if desired.

Variation Tip: I like to substitute spinach for the kale when I'm in the mood.

Per serving (1 cup): Calories: 225, Total Fat: 9g, Saturated Fat: 1g, Cholesterol: 0mg, Sodium: 79mg, Carbohydrates: 27g, Fiber: 9g, Protein: 11g

Quinoa and Greens Soup

GLUTEN-FREE • DAIRY-FREE • NIGHTSHADE-FREE • VEGAN

SERVES 4   **PREP** 5 minutes   **COOK** 25 minutes

I call this a soup, but the quinoa and beans actually create more of a hearty stew. The spinach and squash make for a colorful, appetizing meal that will be a family favorite any night of the week!

2 tablespoons avocado oil

2 medium carrots, chopped

2 celery stalks, chopped

1 medium onion, chopped

3 garlic cloves, chopped

1 yellow squash, diced

1 (15-ounce) can cannellini beans, rinsed and drained

1 cup quinoa, rinsed and drained

½ teaspoon ground cumin

4 cups low-sodium vegetable broth

4 cups spinach

Kosher salt (optional)

Freshly ground black pepper (optional)

1. In a large stockpot over medium heat, warm the avocado oil.

2. Add the carrots, celery, onion, and garlic. Cook until the vegetables are soft, about 10 minutes.

3. Add the squash, beans, quinoa, cumin, broth, and 2 cups water.

4. Bring the mixture to a boil, then reduce the heat to medium and cook until the quinoa is tender, about 13 minutes.

5. Stir in the spinach and cook for about 1 minute, until wilted.

6. Season with salt and pepper, if desired, and serve.

Make It Easier Tip: Use 1 cup chopped frozen carrots and 1½ teaspoons pre-minced garlic instead of fresh.

Per serving (1½ cups): Calories: 364, Total Fat: 10g, Saturated Fat: 1g, Cholesterol: 0mg, Sodium: 148mg, Carbohydrates: 56g, Fiber: 11g, Protein: 16g

Turkey and Cauliflower Rice Soup

GLUTEN-FREE • DAIRY-FREE

SERVES 4   **PREP** 5 minutes   **COOK** 25 minutes

This one-pot recipe delivers on convenience, and the anti-inflammatory turmeric and black pepper give the soup a warming, delicious flavor! This recipe is more filling than your average soup, but you can always add 1 (15-ounce) can black beans for an even heartier version.

2 tablespoons extra-virgin olive oil

1 cup chopped red onion

1 garlic clove, minced

1 pound ground turkey

½ cup chopped carrots

½ tablespoon ground turmeric

¼ teaspoon kosher salt

¼ teaspoon freshly ground black pepper

1 bell pepper, chopped

1 cup riced cauliflower

4 cups low-sodium chicken broth

1. In a large stockpot over medium-high heat, warm the olive oil. Add the onion and garlic and sauté until soft, about 5 minutes.

2. Add the turkey and cook until evenly browned and cooked through, about 8 minutes.

3. Stir in the carrots, turmeric, salt, and black pepper and sauté for 1 more minute.

4. Add the bell pepper, cauliflower, and broth and bring to a boil. Let the mixture boil for about 5 minutes, then serve.

Substitution Tip: If avoiding nightshades, omit the bell pepper and add 1 cup chopped celery.

Ingredient Tip: To make riced cauliflower, roughly chop the cauliflower into florets. Put the florets into a food processor and process until the cauliflower is finely minced into small pieces resembling rice, about 1 minute.

Per serving (1½ cups): Calories: 281, Total Fat: 17g, Saturated Fat: 4g, Cholesterol: 90mg, Sodium: 309mg, Carbohydrates: 10g, Fiber: 2g, Protein: 23g

Cucumber and Avocado Salad

GLUTEN-FREE • DAIRY-FREE • NIGHTSHADE-FREE • VEGAN

SERVES 4 **PREP** 10 minutes

This refreshing salad is the perfect anti-inflammatory side dish, but it can also stand alone as an entrée when served over a bed of fresh greens. Avocados contain healthy monounsaturated fats that help fight inflammation and are high in fiber to feed the gut microbiome.

3 large cucumbers, chopped

1 medium red onion, diced

2 avocados, pitted, peeled, and diced

¼ cup freshly squeezed lemon juice

2 tablespoons extra-virgin olive oil

½ teaspoon kosher salt

⅛ teaspoon freshly ground black pepper

1. In a large bowl, combine the cucumbers, red onion, and avocados.

2. In a small bowl, whisk together the lemon juice, olive oil, salt, and pepper.

3. Pour the dressing over the cucumber mixture and toss gently to coat.

4. Serve immediately.

Variation Tip: If you include nightshades in your meal plan, add some chopped Roma tomatoes for a pop of color.

Per serving (½ cup): Calories: 253, Total Fat: 21g, Saturated Fat: 3g,

Cholesterol: 0mg, Sodium: 250mg, Carbohydrates: 19g, Fiber: 8g, Protein: 4g

Blueberry-Spinach Salad

GLUTEN-FREE · DAIRY-FREE · NIGHTSHADE-FREE · VEGAN

SERVES 2   **PREP** 10 minutes

Blueberries are tiny, but don't let their size fool you! That little package has just the right amount of sweetness but also contains loads of nutrition in the form of antioxidants important for heart, brain, and metabolic health.

6 cups baby spinach

1 cup fresh blueberries

¼ cup chopped walnuts

2 tablespoons sunflower seeds

2 tablespoons avocado oil

2 tablespoons apple cider vinegar (with the mother)

½ teaspoon Dijon mustard

¼ teaspoon kosher salt

⅛ teaspoon freshly ground black pepper

1. In a large bowl, combine the spinach, blueberries, walnuts, and sunflower seeds and mix well.

2. In a small bowl, whisk together the avocado oil, apple cider vinegar, mustard, salt, and pepper.

3. Pour the dressing over the spinach mixture and toss to coat.

4. Serve immediately.

Variation Tip: I like to use a variety of greens in this salad to gain even more nutrient goodness. My favorite mixture includes dandelion greens, kale, arugula, and spinach.

Per serving (about 3 cups): Calories: 342, Total Fat: 29g, Saturated Fat: 3g, Cholesterol: 0mg, Sodium: 321mg, Carbohydrates: 17g, Fiber: 6g, Protein: 7g

Cranberry-Walnut Pear Salad

GLUTEN-FREE • DAIRY-FREE • NIGHTSHADE-FREE • VEGETARIAN

SERVES 2 **PREP** 10 minutes

A peppery Mediterranean green that is a member of the cruciferous vegetable family, arugula is a great way to spice up the average salad. I love the combination of spicy and sweet in this dish, and adding some diced chicken can easily change this from a side salad to a filling entrée.

2 tablespoons extra-virgin olive oil

1 tablespoon apple cider vinegar (with the mother)

½ teaspoon honey

2 cups arugula

1 head Bibb lettuce, chopped

1 pear, cut into thin slices

2 tablespoons dried cranberries

2 tablespoons chopped walnuts

1. In a small bowl, whisk together the olive oil, vinegar, and honey.

2. In a large bowl, combine the arugula and lettuce.

3. Pour the dressing over the lettuce mixture and toss to coat.

4. Top with the pear, cranberries, and walnuts.

Variation Tip: Mix up the combinations of dark leafy greens in this salad. My favorites are dandelion greens and spinach.

Per serving (about 2 cups): Calories: 271, Total Fat: 20g, Saturated Fat: 3g, Cholesterol: 0mg, Sodium: 16mg, Carbohydrates: 24g, Fiber: 4, Protein: 3g

Brussels Sprouts and Broccoli Salad

GLUTEN-FREE • DAIRY-FREE • NIGHTSHADE-FREE • VEGAN

SERVES 6 **PREP** 15 minutes

If you're looking for a go-to potluck dish, this salad is always a crowd-pleaser. The slightly sweet cranberries and crunchy cruciferous vegetables make an unbelievable combination. Hint: This dish always tastes better the next day, so I mix this up the night before and let all the yummy flavors meld overnight before serving.

1 pound Brussels sprouts, trimmed

½ head red cabbage

1 head broccoli, finely chopped

¼ cup dried cranberries

½ cup chopped pecans

½ cup extra-virgin olive oil

¼ cup freshly squeezed lemon juice

4 garlic cloves, chopped

½ cup chopped scallions

¼ teaspoon kosher salt

⅛ teaspoon freshly ground black pepper

1. Put the Brussels sprouts into a food processor and pulse until shredded. Transfer to a large bowl.

2. Put the cabbage into the food processor and pulse until shredded. Add the cabbage to the Brussels sprouts.

3. Add the broccoli, dried cranberries, and pecans and mix well.

4. In a small bowl, whisk together the olive oil, lemon juice, garlic, scallions, salt, and pepper.

5. Pour the dressing over the salad and toss to coat.

Ingredient Tip: I like to slightly steam my Brussels sprouts before shredding them, but they are great raw, too!

Per serving (1 cup): Calories: 293, Total Fat: 24g, Saturated Fat: 3g, Cholesterol: 0mg, Sodium: 132mg, Carbohydrates: 19g, Fiber: 7g, Protein: 6g

Cauliflower Dijon Salad

GLUTEN-FREE • DAIRY-FREE • NIGHTSHADE-FREE • VEGETARIAN

SERVES 4   **PREP** 15 minutes

This flavorful salad is the ideal side dish, but I also like to devour this for breakfast. The tanginess of the tart cherries, Dijon mustard, and apple cider vinegar paired with just a touch of sweetness make this one of my favorites.

1 head cauliflower, cut into bite-size florets

½ cup raw sunflower seeds

½ cup chopped red onion

⅓ cup dried tart cherries

⅓ cup extra-virgin olive oil

2 tablespoons apple cider vinegar (with the mother)

1 tablespoon Dijon mustard

1 tablespoon honey

1 garlic clove, chopped

¼ teaspoon kosher salt

4 cups chopped red leaf lettuce

1. In a large bowl, combine the cauliflower, sunflower seeds, onion, and cherries.

2. In a small bowl, whisk together the olive oil, vinegar, mustard, honey, garlic, and salt.

3. Pour the dressing over the cauliflower mixture and mix well.

4. Divide the lettuce equally among 4 bowls. Top each bowl of lettuce with 1 cup of the cauliflower mixture.

Variation Tip: Instead of sunflower seeds and cherries, try ½ cup chopped pecans and ⅓ cup dried cranberries.

Per serving (1 cup leaf lettuce, 1 cup cauliflower mixture): Calories: 326, Total Fat: 25g, Saturated Fat: 3g, Cholesterol: 0mg, Sodium: 192mg, Carbohydrates: 24g, Fiber: 4g, Protein: 6g

Grilled Chicken and Nectarine Salad

GLUTEN-FREE • DAIRY-FREE • NIGHTSHADE-FREE

SERVES 4   **PREP** 10 minutes   **COOK** 20 minutes

I love adding fruit to salads. The warm, slightly caramelized nectarines in this dish create the perfect explosion of flavor. To complete this meal, add a side of Savory Roasted Herbed Vegetables (page 44).

3 tablespoons extra-virgin olive oil, divided

4 boneless, skinless chicken breasts

¼ teaspoon kosher salt

¼ teaspoon freshly ground black pepper

2 nectarines, pitted and cut into thin slices

2 scallions, chopped

6 cups baby arugula

1 teaspoon dried dill

¼ cup slivered almonds

1. In a large skillet over medium heat, warm 1 tablespoon olive oil.

2. Season the chicken breasts with salt and pepper and, when the oil is hot, add them to the skillet.

3. Cook for 7 minutes on each side, or until the chicken reaches an internal temperature of 165°F. Transfer the chicken to a cutting board.

4. Meanwhile, in a large bowl, combine the nectarines with 1 tablespoon olive oil and toss to coat.

5. Reduce the heat to medium. Using the same skillet, cook the nectarines for 2 minutes on each side.

6. While the nectarines are cooking, dice the chicken.

7. In a large bowl, combine the remaining 1 tablespoon olive oil, chicken, nectarines, scallions, arugula, dill, and almonds and toss. Serve immediately.

Ingredient Tip: Choose nectarines that are brightly colored and slightly soft for the best flavor.

Per serving (about 1½ cups): Calories: 272, Total Fat: 14g, Saturated Fat: 2g, Cholesterol: 65mg, Sodium: 202mg, Carbohydrates: 10g, Fiber: 2g, Protein: 29g

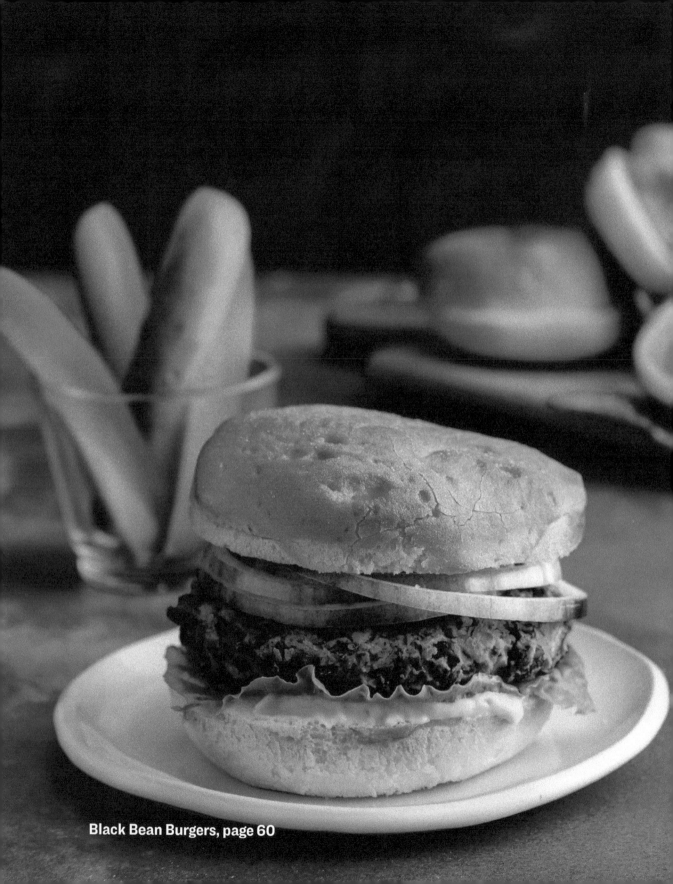

Black Bean Burgers, page 60

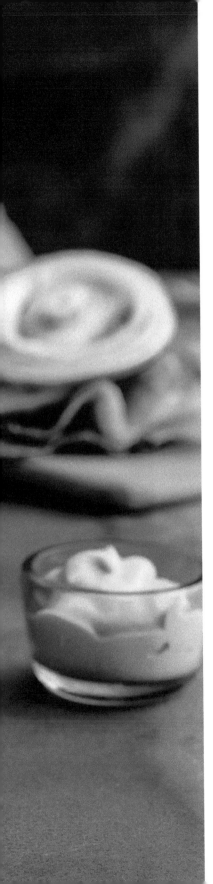

5
VEGETARIAN AND VEGAN

Black Bean Burgers

GLUTEN-FREE • DAIRY-FREE • VEGETARIAN

SERVES 5   **PREP** 10 minutes   **COOK** 15 minutes

When I first made these hearty black bean burgers for my husband, he was definitely skeptical. But once he bit into the crispy outer layer and melty interior, there was no turning back! These are a favorite at our house, and it's my husband who perfected this recipe to create the ultimate plant-based burger.

2 (15-ounce) cans black beans, rinsed, drained, and patted dry (or 1½ cups dried black beans, soaked, rinsed, cooked, and drained)

1 teaspoon paprika

½ teaspoon kosher salt

½ teaspoon freshly ground black pepper

½ teaspoon ground coriander

½ teaspoon ground cumin

1 tablespoon chili powder

1 large egg, beaten

¼ medium red onion, diced

½ jalapeño, diced

1 tablespoon gluten-free oat flour, plus more as needed

2 tablespoons avocado oil

1. In a large bowl, mash the black beans into a paste with a fork.

2. In a small bowl, combine the paprika, salt, pepper, coriander, cumin, and chili powder and mix.

3. Add the seasonings from the small bowl, along with the egg, red onion, and jalapeño, to the black beans and mix well.

4. Add the oat flour to thicken the mixture. (You can add more flour to bring the patties together, if needed.) Shape the mixture into 5 black bean patties.

5. In a large skillet over medium heat, warm the avocado oil. Add the burgers to the skillet and reduce the heat to medium-low.

6. Cook the patties for 7 minutes, then flip and cook for 7 minutes more, or until the exterior reaches your desired crispiness.

7. Serve with your favorite burger toppings.

Substitution Tip: To make these burgers vegan, use an egg replacement like aquafaba (see tip on page 37). Use 3 tablespoons aquafaba for 1 whole large egg. If avoiding nightshades, omit the paprika, chili powder, and jalapeño and increase the cumin to 1 tablespoon.

Per serving (1 patty): Calories: 185, Total Fat: 5g, Saturated Fat: 1g, Cholesterol: 0mg, Sodium: 218mg, Carbohydrates: 26g, Fiber: 10g, Protein: 11g

Zucchini-Bean Bake

GLUTEN-FREE • DAIRY-FREE • NIGHTSHADE-FREE • VEGAN

SERVES 6　**PREP** 10 minutes　**COOK** 40 minutes

Casseroles take the pressure off at mealtime because there's no need to plan a side dish. This all-in-one flavorful recipe has you covered on anti-inflammatory nutrients and fiber.

2 tablespoons coconut oil, divided

2 garlic cloves, chopped

2 (15-ounce) cans black beans, rinsed and drained (or 1½ cups dried black beans soaked, rinsed, cooked, and drained)

1 teaspoon ground cumin

½ teaspoon dried oregano

½ teaspoon dried thyme

1 large zucchini, cut into ¼-inch slices

2 medium yellow squash, cut into ¼-inch slices

2 small red onions, quartered

1½ cups Spinach-Pecan Pesto (page 112)

1. Preheat the oven to 350°F. Line a 9-by-13-inch baking dish with parchment paper.

2. In a large wok or skillet over medium-high heat, warm 1 tablespoon coconut oil. Add the garlic and sauté until fragrant, about 3 minutes.

3. Add the black beans, cumin, oregano, thyme, and ¼ cup water. Cover the skillet, reduce the heat to medium, and cook for 7 minutes, stirring once.

4. Add the remaining 1 tablespoon coconut oil, as well as the zucchini, squash, and onions. Cover and cook until softened, about 10 minutes.

5. Transfer the bean and vegetable mixture to the baking dish.

6. Bake uncovered for 20 minutes.

7. To serve, divide the casserole evenly among 6 bowls and top each portion with ¼ cup spinach-pecan pesto.

Make It Easier Tip: Prepare the spinach-pecan pesto ahead of time and store in the refrigerator to be used in a variety of anti-inflammatory recipes.

Per serving (about 1½ cups): Calories: 312, Total Fat: 19g, Saturated Fat: 6g, Cholesterol: 0mg, Sodium: 77mg, Carbohydrates: 28g, Fiber: 10g, Protein: 10g

Roasted Chickpea Salad

GLUTEN-FREE • DAIRY-FREE • VEGAN

SERVES 2   **PREP** 10 minutes   **COOK** 25 minutes

Chickpeas, also known as garbanzo beans, are a legume high in fiber and protein. They have a nutty flavor and grainy texture and are an awesome meat substitute. I eat the roasted chickpeas in this dish as a snack by themselves, but they are a great addition to any salad as a healthy alternative to croutons.

1 (15-ounce) can chickpeas, rinsed and drained

1 tablespoon avocado oil

1 teaspoon ground cumin

½ teaspoon ground turmeric

½ teaspoon kosher salt

½ teaspoon ground cinnamon

¼ teaspoon ground ginger

6 cups spinach

10 grape tomatoes

½ medium red onion, thinly sliced

¼ cup extra-virgin olive oil

3 garlic cloves, chopped

1 teaspoon dried dill

2 tablespoons freshly squeezed lemon juice

1. Preheat the oven to 450°F. Line a baking sheet with parchment paper.

2. In a medium bowl, combine the chickpeas, avocado oil, cumin, turmeric, salt, cinnamon, and ginger. Mix well.

3. Spread the chickpeas on the baking sheet in a single layer. Bake for 25 minutes, stirring once.

4. While the chickpeas are baking, in a large bowl, combine the spinach, tomatoes, and onion and set aside.

5. In a small bowl, whisk together the olive oil, garlic, dill, and lemon juice.

6. Top the salad with the roasted chickpeas.

7. Pour the dressing over the mixture and toss to coat.

Substitution Tip: If avoiding nightshades, omit the tomatoes and add another of your favorite salad vegetables. Cucumbers would be a great option in this dish.

Per serving (3½ cups salad, ¾ cup chickpeas): Calories: 570, Total Fat: 39g, Saturated Fat: 5g, Cholesterol: 0mg, Sodium: 560mg, Carbohydrates: 46g, Fiber: 14g, Protein: 15g

Mediterranean Lentil Salad

GLUTEN-FREE • DAIRY-FREE • NIGHTSHADE-FREE • VEGAN

SERVES 4   **PREP** 10 minutes   **COOK** 30 minutes

This salad delivers on flavor and nutrition. Olives are a powerful little fruit that provide valuable monoun-saturated fats and antioxidants important for lowering inflammation. Add them to salads, sandwiches, and casseroles or simply eat them by themselves for a filling snack.

1 cup dried brown or green lentils

3 cups spinach

½ medium red onion, sliced

1 medium cucumber, chopped

⅓ cup pitted green olives, chopped

¼ cup extra-virgin olive oil

2 tablespoons balsamic vinegar

2 garlic cloves, chopped

½ teaspoon dried oregano

½ teaspoon dried basil

1. Using a fine-mesh strainer, rinse the lentils.

2. Pour 3 cups water into a medium saucepan. Add the lentils and bring to a boil over medium-high heat.

3. Reduce the heat to low and simmer, stirring occasionally, for about 25 minutes, or until the lentils are tender.

4. While the lentils are cooking, in a large bowl, combine the spinach, onion, cucumber, and olives.

5. In a small bowl, whisk together the olive oil, vinegar, garlic, oregano, and basil.

6. When the lentils are fully cooked, drain and allow to cool.

7. Top the salad with the cooled lentils.

8. Pour the dressing over the mixture and toss to coat.

> **Make It Easier Tip:** Use 1 (15-ounce) can lentils instead of dried lentils and omit steps 1, 2, 3, and 6.

Per serving (about ½ cup lentils, ¾ cup salad mixture): Calories: 323, Total Fat: 15g, Saturated Fat: 2g, Cholesterol: 0mg, Sodium: 323mg, Carbohydrates: 36g, Fiber: 16g, Protein: 14g

Jalapeño Chickpea Spread

GLUTEN-FREE • DAIRY-FREE • VEGAN

SERVES 3   **PREP** 15 minutes

This slightly spicy vegan chickpea spread is the ideal portable lunch option. I love this recipe served in a collard green wrap or as a topper for a mixed green salad.

1 (15-ounce) can chickpeas, rinsed and drained

2 celery stalks, finely chopped

¼ cup chopped red bell pepper

½ jalapeño, chopped

¼ cup extra-virgin olive oil

1 garlic clove, minced

2 teaspoons Dijon mustard

1 tablespoon freshly squeezed lemon juice

¼ teaspoon freshly ground black pepper

1. In a medium bowl, mash the chickpeas into a paste with a fork.

2. Add the celery, bell pepper, and jalapeño and mix until well combined.

3. In a small bowl, whisk together the olive oil, garlic, mustard, lemon juice, and black pepper.

4. Add the dressing to the chickpea mixture and mix well to combine.

Substitution Tip: If avoiding nightshades, omit the jalapeño and bell pepper and replace with ¼ cup each finely chopped onion and carrot.

Per serving (½ cup): Calories: 292, Total Fat: 19g, Saturated Fat: 3g, Cholesterol: 0mg, Sodium: 66mg, Carbohydrates: 25g, Fiber: 7g, Protein: 8g

Quinoa-Veggie Pesto Bowls

GLUTEN-FREE • DAIRY-FREE • VEGAN

SERVES 4   **PREP** 15 minutes   **COOK** 30 minutes

Veggie bowls are a wonderful way to load up on plant-based nutrients with endless combinations. The burst of flavor from the Spinach-Pecan Pesto (page 112) adds the perfect touch to the colorful peppers and cruciferous vegetables in this dish.

½ cup quinoa

2 tablespoons coconut oil

1 head cauliflower, cut into bite-size florets

1 pound Brussels sprouts, trimmed and halved

6 small multicolored mini bell peppers, sliced in half and seeds removed

1 (15-ounce) can Great Northern beans, rinsed and drained

1 avocado, pitted, peeled, and sliced

1 cup Spinach-Pecan Pesto (page 112)

1. Using a fine-mesh strainer, rinse the quinoa.

2. Pour 1 cup water into a small saucepan. Add the quinoa and bring to a boil over medium-high heat. Reduce the heat to low, cover, and cook for 15 minutes. Remove the pot from the heat and let it sit, covered, for 5 minutes.

3. Meanwhile, in a large skillet or wok over medium-high heat, warm the coconut oil. Add the cauliflower, Brussels sprouts, peppers, and beans and stir. Reduce the heat to medium and sauté until the vegetables have softened, about 10 minutes.

4. In each of 4 bowls, put ¼ cup cooked quinoa, ⅓ cup beans, 1 cup vegetables, and ¼ sliced avocado. Drizzle each bowl with ¼ cup pesto.

Substitution Tip: If avoiding nightshades, omit the bell peppers and replace with 1½ cups diced carrots.

Per serving (about ¼ cup quinoa, ⅓ cup beans, 1 cup vegetables, ¼ cup pesto): Calories: 523, Total Fat: 30g, Saturated Fat: 9g, Cholesterol: 0mg, Sodium: 163mg, Carbohydrates: 55g, Fiber: 18g, Protein: 17g

Kale and Chickpea Curry

GLUTEN-FREE • DAIRY-FREE • VEGAN

SERVES 4   **PREP** 10 minutes   **COOK** 30 minutes

This rich, warming one-pot meatless meal is not only high in protein but also delivers about one-third of your daily fiber requirement. It is great served over brown rice and reheats well, making it ideal for batch cooking.

1 tablespoon coconut oil

1 small onion, diced

1 tablespoon curry powder

2 garlic cloves, minced

2 tablespoons fresh grated ginger, or ½ teaspoon ground ginger

1 cup diced sweet potatoes

3 cups small cauliflower florets

¼ teaspoon kosher salt

¼ teaspoon freshly ground black pepper

1 cup low-sodium vegetable broth

1 cup canned chickpeas, rinsed and drained

1 bunch lacinato kale, stems removed and chopped

1. In a large stockpot over medium heat, warm the coconut oil. Add the onion and cook until softened, about 5 minutes.

2. Add the curry powder and cook for 3 more minutes, stirring often.

3. Stir in the garlic and ginger and cook for 2 minutes.

4. Add the sweet potatoes, cauliflower, salt, pepper, and 1 cup water and mix well to combine.

5. Add the broth, cover, and bring to a boil. Reduce the heat to medium-low and simmer for about 15 minutes, or until the potatoes are soft.

6. Add the chickpeas and chopped kale.

7. Simmer for 5 minutes more, or until the greens have wilted.

Ingredient Tip: Many store-bought curry powders contain nightshades, so if you want to avoid nightshades, make your own. Combine 1 teaspoon each of ground turmeric, ground cumin, ground coriander, ground ginger, and dry mustard and ¼ teaspoon each ground cinnamon and black pepper. This will make about 2 tablespoons homemade curry powder. Feel free to use the entire amount in this recipe or save the leftovers in an airtight container for another recipe.

Per serving (1½ cups): Calories: 216, Total Fat: 5g, Saturated Fat: 3g, Cholesterol: 0mg, Sodium: 367mg, Carbohydrates: 36g, Fiber: 8g, Protein: 9g

Kale, Cauliflower, and Quinoa Bowls

GLUTEN-FREE • DAIRY-FREE • NIGHTSHADE-FREE • VEGAN

SERVES 4 **PREP** 5 minutes **COOK** 25 minutes

This recipe highlights kale, a cruciferous vegetable with anti-inflammatory and antioxidant benefits. In addition, this simple, colorful dish is high in protein and the raisins add just the right amount of sweetness.

1 head cauliflower, cut into bite-size florets

2 tablespoons avocado oil

¾ teaspoon kosher salt, divided

¼ teaspoon freshly ground black pepper

¼ cup freshly squeezed lemon juice

3 tablespoons extra-virgin olive oil

1 bunch kale, stems removed and chopped

1 cup cooked quinoa

¼ small red onion, thinly sliced

⅓ cup raisins

⅓ cup sunflower seeds

1. Preheat the oven to 450°F. Line a baking sheet with parchment paper.

2. In a large bowl, combine the cauliflower, avocado oil, ¼ teaspoon salt, and pepper.

3. Place the cauliflower on the baking sheet and bake for 25 minutes, or until tender.

4. In a separate large bowl, whisk together the lemon juice, olive oil, and remaining ½ teaspoon salt.

5. Add the kale and toss until well coated with the dressing.

6. Add the cooked cauliflower, quinoa, onion, raisins, and sunflower seeds and toss to combine.

Make it Easier Tip: Instead of using fresh cauliflower, omit steps 1 and 3 and microwave about 3 cups frozen cauliflower per package instructions. Follow step 2 to season.

Per serving (about 1½ cups): Calories: 366, Total Fat: 24g, Saturated Fat: 3g, Cholesterol: 0mg, Sodium: 144mg, Carbohydrates: 34g, Fiber: 6g, Protein: 8g

Vegan "Meatballs"

GLUTEN-FREE • DAIRY-FREE • NIGHTSHADE-FREE • VEGAN

SERVES 3   **PREP** 10 minutes   **COOK** 20 minutes

Mushrooms have powerful anti-inflammatory and immune-boosting benefits. They can also help improve vitamin D levels, which are routinely inadequate in those with autoimmune diseases like psoriasis. If you're new to trying mushrooms or not much of a mushroom fan, this recipe is the perfect place to start! Try adding Spinach-Pecan Pesto (page 112) as a sauce.

1 (15-ounce) can kidney beans, rinsed and drained

1 tablespoon avocado oil

1 small red onion, chopped

1 garlic clove, chopped

½ cup chopped baby Bella (crimini) mushrooms

1 teaspoon dried oregano

1 teaspoon dried basil

1 tablespoon almond butter

½ cup gluten-free rolled oats

¼ cup whole-milled flaxseed

¼ teaspoon kosher salt

¼ teaspoon freshly ground black pepper

1. Preheat the oven to 350°F. Line a baking sheet with parchment paper.

2. In a medium bowl, mash the kidney beans into a paste with a fork.

3. In a medium skillet over medium heat, heat the oil. Sauté the onion, garlic, and mushrooms for 5 minutes.

4. Add the mushroom mixture to the mashed beans and mix in the oregano, basil, almond butter, and oats.

5. Add the whole-milled flaxseed to the bean mixture and stir until well combined.

6. Season with the salt and pepper.

7. Form the mixture into 12 to 14 balls.

8. Place the balls on the baking sheet and bake for 15 minutes.

Batch Cook Tip: This recipe freezes well, so double the amount and freeze half the "meatballs" for later use.

Per serving (4 meatballs): Calories: 298, Total Fat: 12g, Saturated Fat: 1g, Cholesterol: 0mg, Sodium: 183mg, Carbohydrates: 37g, Fiber: 11g, Protein: 13g

Walnut-Mushroom Burgers

GLUTEN-FREE • DAIRY-FREE • NIGHTSHADE-FREE • VEGAN

SERVES 4   **PREP** 10 minutes   **COOK** 35 minutes, plus 2 hours to chill

This recipe is another wonderful way to include more mushrooms in your meal plan. Of course, you can eat mushrooms raw on salads, but they are also great incorporated into a variety of cooked recipes, such as these walnut-mushroom burgers, which are guaranteed to be a family favorite! These burgers reheat well, making them a perfect option for lunch the next day.

4 medium portobello mushroom caps (about 1 pound), gills removed, chopped

½ cup chopped walnuts

1 garlic clove, chopped

1 tablespoon extra-virgin olive oil

¼ teaspoon kosher salt

¼ teaspoon freshly ground black pepper

¼ cup chopped red onion

3 scallions, chopped

2 teaspoons red wine vinegar

1 cup cooked quinoa

½ cup gluten-free oat flour

1 tablespoon avocado oil

1. Preheat the oven to 375°F. Line a rimmed baking sheet with parchment paper.

2. In a medium bowl, combine the mushrooms, walnuts, garlic, olive oil, salt, and pepper and mix well.

3. Spread the mixture on the baking sheet in an even layer and bake for 20 minutes, or until the mushrooms are tender.

4. Remove from the oven and allow the mushrooms to cool.

5. Put the cooked mushrooms, onion, scallions, and vinegar into a food processor and pulse until smooth. Transfer the mixture to a large bowl.

6. Stir in the quinoa and oat flour until well combined. Cover the mixture and refrigerate for 2 hours.

7. Preheat the oven to 375°F. Line a baking sheet with parchment paper.

8. Divide the mushroom mixture into 4 equal portions, forming each portion into a patty.

9. In a large skillet over medium heat, warm the avocado oil.

10. Place the patties in the skillet and cook for 2 minutes on each side, or until browned.

11. Transfer the browned patties to the parchment-lined baking sheet and bake in the oven for 10 minutes.

12. Serve with your favorite burger toppings.

Make Ahead Tip: Make the recipe through step 8 the day before to save time.

Per serving (1 patty): Calories: 305, Total Fat: 19g, Saturated Fat: 2g,

Cholesterol: 0mg, Sodium: 128mg, Carbohydrates: 26g, Fiber: 6g, Protein: 9g

Black Bean–Tofu Bowls

GLUTEN-FREE • DAIRY-FREE • VEGAN

SERVES 4   **PREP** 10 minutes   **COOK** 15 minutes

Tofu is a nutrient-dense, plant-based complete protein. It can be used in a variety of recipes, has a very mild flavor, and is a great meat alternative.

1 tablespoon avocado oil

1 red onion, chopped

3 garlic cloves, chopped

1 (15-ounce) can black beans, rinsed and drained

2 teaspoons ground cumin

¼ cup freshly squeezed lime juice, plus more for serving

1 package firm tofu, rinsed and chopped into 1-inch cubes

1 tablespoon extra-virgin olive oil

2 teaspoons smoked paprika

¼ teaspoon kosher salt

¼ teaspoon freshly ground black pepper

1 cup cooked brown rice

2 small ripe avocados, pitted, peeled, and chopped

1. Preheat the oven to broil. Line a baking sheet with parchment paper.

2. In a large skillet over medium heat, warm the avocado oil. Add the onion and garlic and sauté for 5 minutes, or until the onion has softened.

3. Stir in the black beans and cumin. Cover and cook for 5 minutes more.

4. Stir in the lime juice.

5. While the bean mixture cooks, in a medium bowl, gently toss the tofu with the olive oil, paprika, salt, and pepper.

6. Place the tofu on the baking sheet and broil until browned.

7. In each of 4 bowls, put ½ cup black beans, ½ cup tofu, ¼ cup brown rice, and ½ avocado.

8. Drizzle with more lime juice, if desired.

Substitution Tip: If avoiding nightshades, replace the smoked paprika with 2 teaspoons ground cumin.

Per serving (1 bowl): Calories: 416, Total Fat: 25g, Saturated Fat: 4g, Cholesterol: 0mg, Sodium: 139mg, Carbohydrates: 39g, Fiber: 14g, Protein: 16g

Spaghetti Squash Pesto "Pasta"

GLUTEN-FREE • DAIRY-FREE • NIGHTSHADE-FREE • VEGAN

SERVES 2   **PREP** 10 minutes   **COOK** 50 minutes

Sometimes you just want a pasta dish. This recipe fits that bill without the tomato sauce, for those of us avoiding nightshades, and also cuts out the refined carbohydrates found in traditional pasta. With this dish, you will never miss either one!

3 tablespoons extra-virgin olive oil, divided

1 teaspoon ground turmeric

¼ teaspoon kosher salt

¼ teaspoon freshly ground black pepper

1 large spaghetti squash, halved lengthwise and seeded

1 (15-ounce) can chickpeas, rinsed and drained

⅔ cup Spinach-Pecan Pesto (page 112)

1. Preheat the oven to 400°F. Line a baking sheet with parchment paper.

2. In a small bowl, combine 2 tablespoons olive oil with the turmeric, salt, and pepper.

3. Using a pastry brush, coat the interior of the squash with the olive oil mixture and place each half, cut-side down, on the baking sheet.

4. Roast for 45 minutes, or until a knife easily pierces the skin and flesh. Remove the squash from the oven and allow to cool.

5. When cool, use a fork to scrape out the flesh into long, spaghetti-like tendrils.

6. In a medium skillet over medium heat, warm the remaining 1 tablespoon olive oil. Sauté the chickpeas for 5 minutes.

7. Divide the squash between 2 bowls, then top with half the chickpeas and ⅓ cup spinach-pecan pesto.

Make It Easier Tip: To reduce prep time right before dinner, roast the spaghetti squash and make the pesto the night before, then store them in the refrigerator. Simply reheat the squash in a skillet with 1 tablespoon avocado oil.

Per serving (2 cups spaghetti squash with pesto, ¾ cup chickpeas):
Calories: 634, Total Fat: 44g, Saturated Fat: 7g, Cholesterol: 0mg,
Sodium: 369mg, Carbohydrates: 53g, Fiber: 11g, Protein: 14g

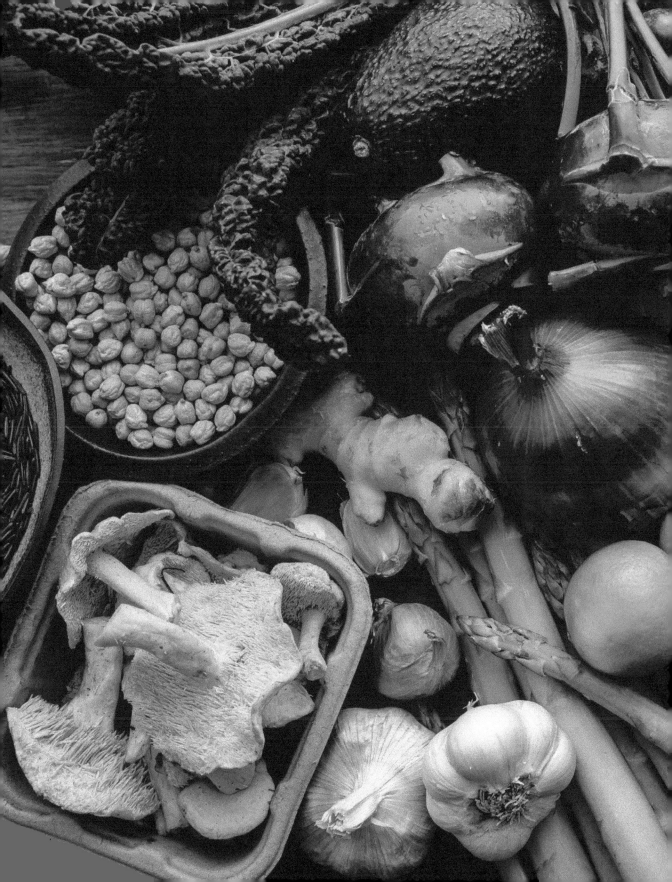

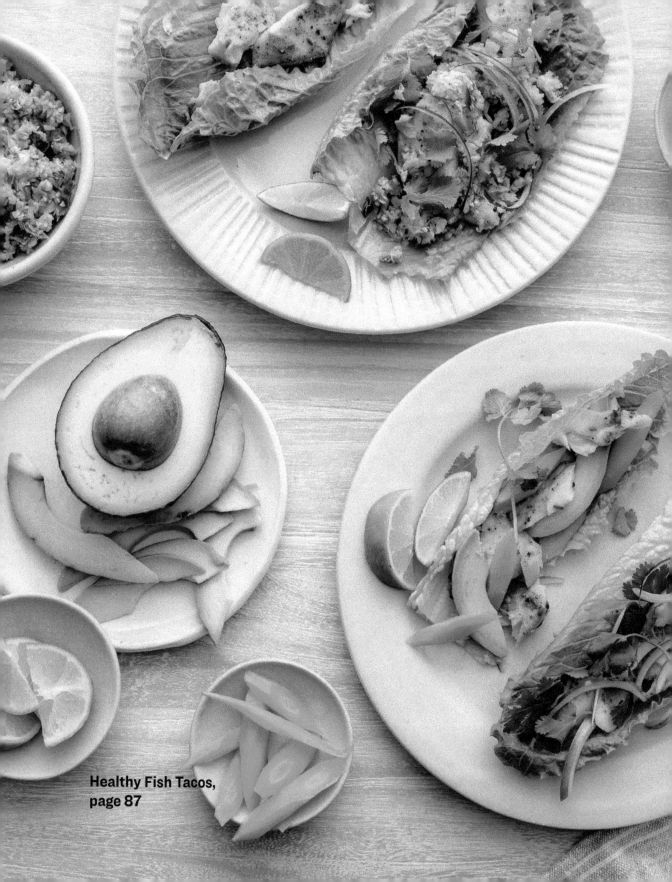

**Healthy Fish Tacos,
page 87**

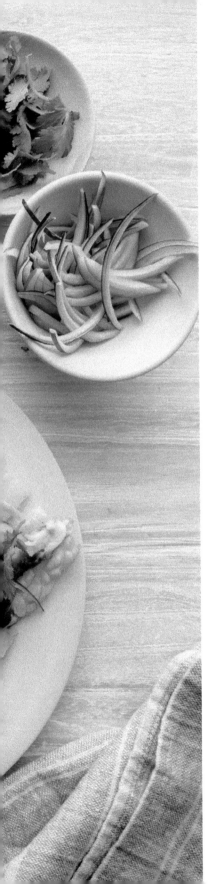

6

FISH AND SEAFOOD

Avocado Tuna Salad

GLUTEN-FREE • DAIRY-FREE • NIGHTSHADE-FREE

SERVES 2   **PREP** 5 minutes

Boring lunches will be a thing of the past with this creamy avocado tuna salad. Tuna is a great source of anti-inflammatory omega-3 fatty acids, and it is also full of lean protein. Instead of the traditional mayonnaise dressing, I use an avocado spread to add healthy fat and fiber, making this a delicious, filling lunch option.

1 ripe avocado, pitted, peeled, and chopped

½ teaspoon kosher salt

Juice of 1 lime

1 tablespoon finely chopped red onion

1 (5-ounce) can light tuna packed in water, drained

Mixed greens or gluten-free wraps, for serving (optional)

1. In a small bowl, mash together the avocado, salt, and lime juice.

2. Add the onion and mix well.

3. Mix in the tuna.

4. Serve atop a fresh bed of greens or in a gluten-free wrap, if desired.

Variation Tip: Add 1 tablespoon chopped fresh dill for a more vibrant flavor.

Per serving (¾ cup): Calories: 208, Total Fat: 14g, Saturated Fat: 2g, Cholesterol: 38mg, Sodium: 673mg, Carbohydrates: 10g, Fiber: 6g, Protein: 15g

Grilled Salmon with Kale and White Beans

GLUTEN-FREE • DAIRY-FREE • NIGHTSHADE-FREE

SERVES 4 **PREP** 10 minutes **COOK** 10 minutes

The light, slightly tangy dressing in this dish balances the stronger flavor of the salmon for a perfect nutrient-dense dinner or leftover lunch. If you prefer to forgo the grill, heat 1 tablespoon coconut oil in a large skillet over medium heat in step 1 and then proceed with the recipe as instructed.

3 tablespoons freshly squeezed lemon juice

2 tablespoons extra-virgin olive oil

1 garlic clove, minced

¾ teaspoon kosher salt

⅛ teaspoon freshly ground black pepper

4 (6-ounce) salmon fillets, with skin

4 cups chopped kale

1 (15-ounce) can Great Northern beans, rinsed and drained

1 red onion, sliced

1. Preheat the grill to medium-high.

2. In a medium bowl, whisk together the lemon juice, olive oil, garlic, salt, and black pepper. Set aside.

3. Place the salmon, skin-side down, on the grill and cook for 6 minutes.

4. Meanwhile, in a large bowl, combine the kale, beans, onion, and lemon-garlic dressing and mix well.

5. Flip the salmon and cook for 4 minutes more, or until each fillet reaches an internal temperature of 145°F.

6. Divide the kale and bean mixture among 4 plates, then top each portion with a cooked salmon fillet.

Variation Tip: Mix up the greens in this recipe by using 2 cups arugula and 2 cups spinach instead of the kale for a slightly different flavor profile.

Per serving (1 salmon fillet, 1½ cups bean-kale mixture): Calories: 351, Total Fat: 10g, Saturated Fat: 1g, Cholesterol: 98mg, Sodium: 580mg, Carbohydrates: 24g, Fiber: 7g, Protein: 43g

Sheet-Pan Miso Salmon and Squash

GLUTEN-FREE • DAIRY-FREE • NIGHTSHADE-FREE

SERVES 4 **PREP** 10 minutes **COOK** 35 minutes

The marinade for the vegetables uses white miso—a food made from fermented soybeans with a sweet, mild flavor—and accented with citrus juices to create a mouthwatering flavor. Use this marinade as a dressing in a variety of recipes.

1 butternut squash, peeled, seeded, and cut into 1-inch cubes

1 large zucchini, cut into 1-inch pieces

1 small head broccoli, cut into bite-size florets

1 medium red onion, cut in half and then quartered

5 tablespoons extra-virgin olive oil, divided, plus more for drizzling

¼ teaspoon kosher salt

1 (1-pound) boneless salmon fillet

¼ cup freshly squeezed orange juice

2 tablespoons freshly squeezed lemon juice

2 tablespoons red wine vinegar

2 tablespoons white miso

1 tablespoon honey

⅓ cup raw pepitas, for topping

1. Preheat the oven to 425°F. Line a baking sheet with parchment paper.

2. In a large bowl, combine the squash, zucchini, broccoli, onion, 3 tablespoons olive oil, and salt. Mix well. Spread the squash mixture on the baking sheet in a single layer and roast for 20 minutes, or until fork-tender.

3. Reduce the oven temperature to 325°F.

4. Arrange the salmon fillet on top of the roasted vegetables. (You can drizzle some olive oil over top at this point, if desired.) Bake for 12 to 15 minutes, or until the salmon reaches an internal temperature of 145°F.

5. Meanwhile, in a small bowl, whisk together the orange and lemon juices, vinegar, miso, honey, and remaining 2 tablespoons olive oil.

6. Cut the cooked salmon into 4 equal portions. Divide the roasted vegetables among 4 plates and top each portion with a piece of salmon.

7. Top each plate with 2 tablespoons of the miso-citrus dressing and a sprinkle of pepitas.

Ingredient Tip: Miso paste can be found in the refrigerated section of most grocery stores, as well as in Asian markets and online.

Per serving (4 ounces salmon, 1½ cups vegetables): Calories: 519, Total Fat: 30g, Saturated Fat: 5g, Cholesterol: 66mg, Sodium: 628mg, Carbohydrates: 40g, Fiber: 8g, Protein: 30g

Crab-Stuffed Avocados

GLUTEN-FREE • DAIRY-FREE • NIGHTSHADE-FREE

SERVES 4   **PREP** 5 minutes   **COOK** 10 minutes

Crab is another great source of anti-inflammatory nutrients such as selenium and omega-3 fatty acids. Pairing crab with the avocado creates a delicate, slightly sweet dish that's high in fiber and full of flavor.

½ cup extra-virgin olive oil

¼ cup freshly squeezed lemon juice

3 teaspoons dried dill

½ teaspoon freshly ground black pepper

2 (8-ounce) cans crabmeat

1 tablespoon avocado oil

2 ripe avocados, pitted, peeled, halved, and partially hollowed out

1. In a medium bowl, whisk together the olive oil, lemon juice, dill, and pepper.

2. Add the crabmeat and mix well.

3. Put the crab mixture in a medium skillet over medium heat and heat through, about 5 minutes. Remove from the skillet and set aside.

4. In the same skillet, heat the avocado oil. Add the avocado halves, cut-side down, and cook for about 2 minutes, or until lightly browned.

5. To serve, spoon about ½ cup crabmeat mixture into each avocado half.

Ingredient Tip: You will need to partially hollow out the avocado to make room for the crabmeat, but save the leftover avocado to add to a salad or freeze it to add to your morning smoothie.

Per serving (½ avocado): Calories: 499, Total Fat: 44g, Saturated Fat: 6g, Cholesterol: 61mg, Sodium: 720mg, Carbohydrates: 10g, Fiber: 6g, Protein: 16g

Italian Fish Cakes

GLUTEN-FREE • DAIRY-FREE • NIGHTSHADE-FREE

SERVES 3 **PREP** 5 minutes **COOK** 15 minutes

As a kid, I always loved my mom's fried fish cakes. Instead of deep-frying the fish cakes, this gluten-free recipe starts with a short panfry on the stove to create that delicious crispy outer layer, before finishing in the oven to result in a warm, flaky center. Complete your meal with Simple Turmeric Roasted Carrots (page 40) and Creamy Cauliflower Mash (page 41).

12 ounces skinless halibut fillets, cut into ½-inch chunks

⅓ cup chopped scallions

¼ cup gluten-free oat flour

1 large egg white

2 garlic cloves

1 teaspoon dried basil

1 teaspoon dried oregano

1 teaspoon ground ginger

2 teaspoons avocado oil

Kosher salt, for serving (optional)

1. Preheat the oven to 350°F.

2. Put the halibut, scallions, oat flour, egg white, garlic, basil, oregano, and ginger in a food processor and pulse until coarsely ground (do not overprocess).

3. Divide the fish mixture into 6 equal portions and form the patties.

4. In a large oven-safe skillet over medium-high heat, warm the avocado oil.

5. Add the patties and cook for 2 to 4 minutes on each side, or until lightly browned.

6. Transfer the skillet to the oven and bake for about 5 minutes.

7. Before serving, sprinkle each fish cake with a dash of salt, if desired.

Substitution Tip: If avoiding eggs, omit the egg white and substitute 2 tablespoons aquafaba (see tip on page 37) liquid.

Per serving (2 fish cakes): Calories: 192, Total Fat: 6g, Saturated Fat: 1g, Cholesterol: 36mg, Sodium: 90mg, Carbohydrates: 8g, Fiber: 2g, Protein: 26g

Halibut with Carrots and Leeks

GLUTEN-FREE • DAIRY-FREE

SERVES 4 **PREP** 10 minutes **COOK** 15 minutes

This quick all-in-one meal is perfect for those hectic weeknights when you just want a simple, delicious dinner with minimal cleanup. Leeks are a member of the same family as onions and garlic and serve as prebiotics to keep the gut microbiome healthy. They have a mild, unique flavor and can be chopped and added raw into salads, used as a base for soups or stews, or enjoyed sautéed as a side dish. To clean the leeks for this recipe, remove the root end and cut the white and light green parts into rings, then soak the rings in cold water and let the dirt and sand from between the layers sink to the bottom. Remove the leeks from the water with a fine-mesh strainer.

1 (14.5-ounce) can sliced carrots, drained

2 cups leeks (about 2 large leeks), cut into rings

1 teaspoon smoked paprika

1 garlic clove, minced

1 teaspoon ground cumin

¼ cup extra-virgin olive oil

¼ teaspoon kosher salt

¼ teaspoon freshly ground black pepper

4 (6-ounce) halibut fillets

1. Preheat the oven to 450°F. Cut 4 (12-by-12-inch) squares of aluminum foil.

2. In a large bowl, mix together the carrots, leeks, paprika, garlic, cumin, olive oil, salt, and pepper.

3. Place 1 cup of the vegetable mixture in the center of each foil square.

4. Place a halibut fillet on top of each portion of vegetables and season with additional salt and pepper, if desired.

5. Seal the foil packets by bringing the sides up to meet at the top, folding the foil lightly to allow room for the steam to gather and cook the fish.

6. Put the packets on a baking sheet and bake for about 15 minutes, or until the fish reaches an internal temperature of 145°F.

Substitution Tip: If avoiding nightshades, omit the paprika and increase the amount of black pepper to 1¼ teaspoons.

Per serving (1 packet): Calories: 358, Total Fat: 17g, Saturated Fat: 3g, Cholesterol: 55mg, Sodium: 290mg, Carbohydrates: 17g, Fiber: 4g, Protein: 37g

Mediterranean Roasted Cod

GLUTEN-FREE • DAIRY-FREE • NIGHTSHADE-FREE

SERVES 4   **PREP** 5 minutes   **COOK** 25 minutes

Bake fish Mediterranean-style with these vibrant flavors: the olives and scallions pair well with the delicate, mild cod to create a tasty anti-inflammatory dish. Complete your meal by adding a side of Cucumber and Avocado Salad (page 52).

2 (15-ounce) cans cannellini beans, rinsed and drained

½ cup pitted olives, chopped

1 teaspoon dried oregano

½ teaspoon kosher salt

¼ teaspoon freshly ground black pepper

1 (1½-pound) whole, skinless cod fillet

2 scallions, chopped

5 tablespoons extra-virgin olive oil

1. Preheat the oven to 300°F.

2. In a large bowl, combine the beans, olives, oregano, salt, pepper, and ½ cup water.

3. Spread the bean mixture in an even layer in a 9-by-13-inch baking dish.

4. Place the cod on top of the bean mixture and season with additional salt and pepper, if desired.

5. Sprinkle the scallions over the fish and drizzle with the olive oil.

6. Bake for 25 minutes, or until the cod reaches an internal temperature of 145°F.

Ingredient Tip: Choose cod that has firm, white flesh and no dark spots.

Per serving (¾ cup bean mixture, 6 ounces cod): Calories: 508, Total Fat: 22g, Saturated Fat: 3g, Cholesterol: 80mg, Sodium: 635mg, Carbohydrates: 36g, Fiber: 11g, Protein: 41g

The Perfect Cod

GLUTEN-FREE • DAIRY-FREE

SERVES 2   **PREP** 5 minutes   **COOK** 20 minutes

Cod has a mild flavor and is a great source of lean protein, so it's the perfect lunch option to keep you alert for the afternoon. This simple yet flavorful cod is the ideal topper for the Blueberry-Spinach Salad (page 53). To make nightshade-free curry powder, see the tip on page 66.

2 (6-ounce) skinless, boneless cod fillets

2 tablespoons extra-virgin olive oil

½ teaspoon kosher salt

2 tablespoons avocado oil

2 garlic cloves, chopped

2 teaspoons Dijon mustard

1 tablespoon ground ginger

2 teaspoons curry powder

1. Preheat the oven to 325°F. Line a baking sheet with parchment paper.

2. Coat the fillets with the olive oil, season them with salt, and place them on the baking sheet.

3. Bake for 12 to 15 minutes, or until the cod reaches an internal temperature of 145°F.

4. Meanwhile, in a small skillet over medium heat, warm the avocado oil. Add the garlic and cook until fragrant, about 3 minutes.

5. Add the mustard, ginger, and curry powder and mix well. Remove from the heat.

6. To serve, drizzle each fillet with half of the mustard sauce.

Variation Tip: For a slightly sweeter version, add 1 tablespoon honey to the mustard sauce.

Per serving (1 cod fillet): Calories: 432, Total Fat: 30g, Saturated Fat: 4g, Cholesterol: 80mg, Sodium: 527mg, Carbohydrates: 8g, Fiber: 1g, Protein: 29g

Italian Baked Tilapia

GLUTEN-FREE • DAIRY-FREE • NIGHTSHADE-FREE

SERVES 4 **PREP** 5 minutes **COOK** 15 minutes

Tilapia, with its mild flavor, allows the Italian seasonings to take center stage in this delicious recipe. I like to serve this alongside the Brussels Sprouts and Broccoli Salad (page 55). For best results, allow the tilapia to marinate in the dressing for 15 to 30 minutes before baking.

4 (6-ounce) tilapia fillets

3 tablespoons extra-virgin olive oil

1 tablespoon freshly squeezed lemon juice

1½ teaspoons garlic powder

½ teaspoon dried oregano

½ teaspoon dried thyme

½ teaspoon dried basil

⅛ teaspoon kosher salt

1. Preheat the oven to 425°F.

2. Place the tilapia fillets in an 8-by-8-inch baking dish.

3. In a small bowl, whisk together the olive oil, lemon juice, garlic powder, oregano, thyme, basil, and salt.

4. Pour the dressing over the tilapia.

5. Bake uncovered for 12 to 15 minutes, or until the tilapia reaches an internal temperature of 145°F.

Ingredient Tip: Tilapia is generally farm-raised, and the safety and quality depends on farming practices. It's best to avoid tilapia sourced from China. Check out SeafoodWatch.org to learn more about sustainable, safe sources of tilapia. If you have difficulty finding safe tilapia, you can substitute an equal amount of salmon or trout in this recipe.

Per serving (1 fillet): Calories: 235, Total Fat: 12g, Saturated Fat: 2g, Cholesterol: 83mg, Sodium: 120mg, Carbohydrates: 1g, Fiber: 0g, Protein: 32g

Healthy Fish Tacos

GLUTEN-FREE · DAIRY-FREE

SERVES 3   **PREP** 5 minutes, plus 30 minutes to marinate   **COOK** 10 minutes

Why wait for Taco Tuesday when these simple, flavorful tacos can be served any night of the week? Pairing mild tilapia with Tangy Coleslaw (page 114) is the perfect combination for a delicious burst of flavor!

1 tablespoon avocado oil

½ teaspoon ground cumin

½ teaspoon chili powder

½ teaspoon onion powder

½ teaspoon garlic powder

1 teaspoon kosher salt

¼ teaspoon freshly ground black pepper

¼ cup freshly squeezed lime juice

1 (1-pound) tilapia fillet

Tangy Coleslaw (page 114), for serving

6 romaine lettuce leaves, for serving

1. In a small bowl, whisk together the avocado oil, cumin, chili powder, onion powder, garlic powder, salt, pepper, and lime juice. Place the tilapia in a shallow dish and cover with the marinade. Cover the dish and let it marinate in the refrigerator for 30 minutes.

2. Preheat the oven to 400°F. Line a baking sheet with parchment paper.

3. Place the marinated fish on the baking sheet and bake for 10 minutes, or until the tilapia reaches an internal temperature of 145°F.

4. Remove from the oven and, using two forks, break the tilapia into flakes.

5. To serve, put the desired amount of the tilapia mixture (about 2 ounces or ¼ cup) on a lettuce leaf, top with 2 tablespoons tangy coleslaw, wrap, and enjoy!

Substitution Tip: If avoiding nightshades, omit the chili powder and increase the amount of cumin to 1 teaspoon.

Per serving (2 fish tacos): Calories: 322, Total Fat: 19g, Saturated Fat: 2g, Cholesterol: 74mg, Sodium: 672mg, Carbohydrates: 11g, Fiber: 3g, Protein: 30g

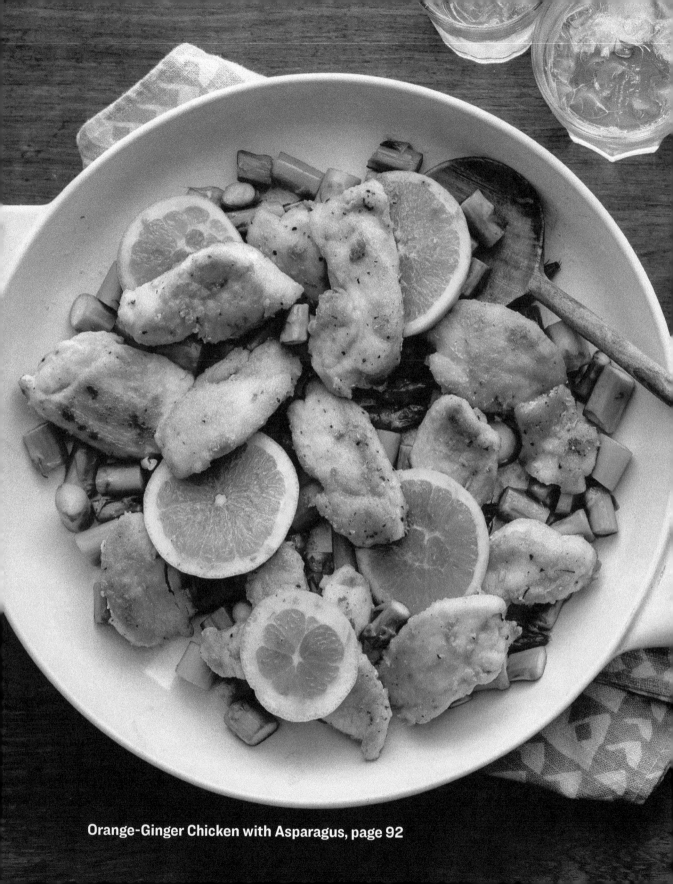

Orange-Ginger Chicken with Asparagus, page 92

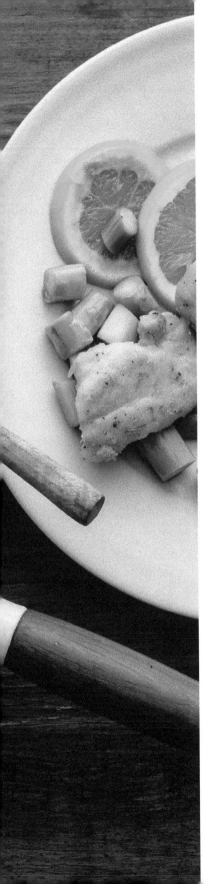

7

POULTRY AND MEAT

Hearty Chicken Casserole

GLUTEN-FREE • DAIRY-FREE • NIGHTSHADE-FREE

SERVES 4 to 6   **PREP** 10 minutes   **COOK** 65 minutes

There's no need to worry about planning lunch when you've got this recipe in the rotation. The finished product is a one-pot nutritious dish that's perfect for family functions but also works well for batch cooking.

1 cup uncooked wild rice

2 tablespoons avocado oil, divided

1 pound boneless, skinless chicken breasts

¼ teaspoon kosher salt

¼ teaspoon freshly ground black pepper

½ medium onion, chopped

1 sweet potato, cubed

1 head broccoli, coarsely chopped

2 garlic cloves, minced

½ teaspoon paprika

½ teaspoon ground cumin

½ cup low-sodium chicken broth, divided

¼ cup dried cranberries

¼ cup walnuts, diced

1. Preheat the oven to 350°F.

2. Put the rice and 2 cups water in a medium saucepan. Bring to a boil, then cover, reduce the heat to low, and simmer for 15 minutes. Remove from the heat and let the pot sit, covered, for 5 minutes.

3. While the rice cooks, in a large skillet over medium heat, warm 1 tablespoon avocado oil. Add the chicken and season with the salt and pepper. Cook for about 8 minutes on each side, or until the chicken has reached an internal temperature of 165°F. Remove from the heat and let cool.

4. While the chicken cooks, in a separate large skillet over medium heat, warm the remaining 1 tablespoon avocado oil. Add the onion, sweet potato, broccoli, garlic, paprika, and cumin.

5. Sauté, stirring regularly, for about 5 minutes, or until the vegetables have softened. Add ¼ cup broth, reduce the heat to low, cover, and simmer for 5 minutes.

6. When the chicken has cooled, cut it into ½-inch cubes.

7. In a large bowl, mix together the cooked rice, chicken, cranberries, and vegetable mixture. Transfer everything to a 9-by-13-inch baking dish.

8. Add the remaining ¼ cup chicken broth and top with the walnuts.

9. Bake for 15 minutes.

Substitution Tip: For a lower-carbohydrate version, substitute 3 cups riced cauliflower for the wild rice in step 7 and omit step 2.

Per serving (about 2 cups): Calories: 454, Total Fat: 14g, Saturated Fat: 1g, Cholesterol: 65mg, Sodium: 239mg, Carbohydrates: 49g, Fiber: 6g, Protein: 36g

Orange-Ginger Chicken with Asparagus

GLUTEN-FREE • DAIRY-FREE • NIGHTSHADE-FREE

SERVES 4   **PREP** 10 minutes   **COOK** 25 minutes

Asparagus is a nutrient-dense, anti-inflammatory vegetable that can be green, white, or purple. Its mild, earthy flavor pairs nicely with ginger and citrus, and the combination will fill your kitchen with the perfect aroma to entice your taste buds.

¼ cup gluten-free oat flour

2 tablespoons minced fresh ginger, or ½ teaspoon ground ginger

¼ teaspoon kosher salt

¼ teaspoon freshly ground black pepper

1 pound boneless, skinless chicken breasts, thinly sliced

2 tablespoons coconut oil, divided

2 cups chopped asparagus

1 orange, cut into thin rings

1. In a shallow dish, combine the oat flour, ginger, salt, and pepper and mix well. Coat each side of the chicken with the mixture.

2. In a large skillet over medium-high heat, warm 1 tablespoon coconut oil.

3. Add the chicken and sauté for 5 minutes on each side.

4. In a separate large skillet over medium-high heat, heat the remaining 1 tablespoon coconut oil.

5. Add the chopped asparagus and sauté for about 5 minutes, or until slightly tender.

6. Add the cooked chicken to the asparagus and layer with the orange rings.

7. Reduce the heat to medium, cover, and cook for 7 minutes, or until the chicken reaches an internal temperature of 165°F.

8. Remove and discard the orange rings before serving.

> **Ingredient Tip:** When shopping for asparagus, make sure the stems are firm and the tips are closed.

Per serving (1 chicken breast, ½ cup asparagus): Calories: 241, Total Fat: 9g, Saturated Fat: 6g, Cholesterol: 65mg, Sodium: 194mg, Carbohydrates: 13g, Fiber: 3g, Protein: 29g

Sheet-Pan Honey Chicken with Brussels Sprouts

GLUTEN-FREE • DAIRY-FREE • NIGHTSHADE-FREE

SERVES 4   **PREP** 10 minutes   **COOK** 25 minutes

Convenience in the kitchen is one of my main priorities, especially on hectic weeknights. This sheet-pan recipe comes together in a flash and highlights the daikon radish, a root vegetable typically used in Japanese cooking. The combination of the slightly sweet, zesty taste of the radish with the more muted flavor of the Brussels sprouts is sure to satisfy.

1 tablespoon extra-virgin olive oil

1 tablespoon honey

1½ tablespoons red wine vinegar

½ tablespoon Dijon mustard

½ teaspoon garlic powder

1 teaspoon dried thyme

½ teaspoon kosher salt

½ teaspoon freshly ground black pepper

1 pound boneless, skinless chicken breasts, cut into 1-inch cubes

½ pound Brussels sprouts, trimmed

1 daikon radish, diced

2 large carrots, cut into 1-inch rounds

1 small onion, chopped

1 medium sweet potato, cut into chunks

1. Preheat the oven to 450°F. Line a baking sheet with parchment paper.

2. In a small bowl, whisk together the olive oil, honey, vinegar, mustard, garlic powder, thyme, salt, and pepper.

3. In a large bowl, combine the chicken and Brussels sprouts, radish, carrots, onion, and sweet potato.

4. Drizzle the dressing over the mixture and stir well to coat.

5. Spread the chicken and vegetables out on the baking sheet and bake for 15 minutes.

6. Stir and flip the meat and vegetables once, then cook for 10 more minutes.

Make It Easier Tip: Prepare all your vegetables and chicken the day before—put them in a large sealable plastic bag with the marinade and store in the refrigerator overnight.

Per serving (about 1½ cups): Calories: 233, Total Fat: 5g, Saturated Fat: 1g, Cholesterol: 65mg, Sodium: 390mg, Carbohydrates: 20g, Fiber: 4g, Protein: 28g

Ginger Chicken Meatballs

GLUTEN-FREE • DAIRY-FREE • NIGHTSHADE-FREE

SERVES 4   **PREP** 5 minutes   **COOK** 15 minutes

Coriander is a spice made from the dried seeds of cilantro and is used in a variety of dishes for its mild, citrusy flavor. Combining coriander and ginger creates tasty anti-inflammatory meatballs that pair well with a variety of dishes. I love adding these to Spaghetti Squash with Broccoli (page 43) or smothering them with Velvety Turmeric Sauce (page 115).

1 pound ground chicken

1 tablespoon ground ginger

1 tablespoon ground coriander

½ teaspoon kosher salt

1 tablespoon coconut oil

1. In a large bowl, mix together the ground chicken, ginger, coriander, and salt.

2. Form the mixture into 16 equal-size meatballs.

3. In a large skillet over medium heat, warm the coconut oil. Gently place the meatballs in the skillet, cover, and cook for 10 minutes, rotating the meatballs frequently until they reach an internal temperature of 165°F. (Total cooking time may be up to 15 minutes.)

Batch Cook Tip: Double the recipe and freeze the leftovers for a quick protein-packed meal option. Simply pull them out of the freezer, thaw in the microwave or the refrigerator, and reheat to an internal temperature of 165°F.

Per serving (4 meatballs): Calories: 194, Total Fat: 13g, Saturated Fat: 6g, Cholesterol: 96mg, Sodium: 302mg, Carbohydrates: 1g, Fiber: 0g, Protein: 20g

Balsamic Chicken

GLUTEN-FREE • DAIRY-FREE • NIGHTSHADE-FREE

SERVES 4   **PREP** 5 minutes   **COOK** 20 minutes

I absolutely love this simple, mouthwatering chicken recipe. Round out your meal with a side of Wilted Swiss Chard with Red Onion and Garlic (page 42) and Creamy Cauliflower Mash (page 41). Any leftover chicken can be chopped and added to a salad for a wholesome lunch.

¼ cup extra-virgin olive oil

2 tablespoons balsamic vinegar

1 tablespoon honey

½ teaspoon dried oregano

½ teaspoon dried thyme

½ teaspoon dried basil

2 tablespoons coconut oil

1 pound chicken breast tenderloins

1. In a large bowl, whisk together the olive oil, vinegar, honey, oregano, thyme, and basil.

2. Add the chicken to the marinade and coat well.

3. In a large skillet over medium heat, warm the coconut oil. Add the marinated chicken.

4. Cook the tenderloins for 8 minutes on each side, or until the chicken reaches an internal temperature of 165°F.

Make it Easier Tip: Marinate the chicken overnight in the refrigerator in a sealed container.

Per serving (3 tenderloins): Calories: 305, Total Fat: 21g, Saturated Fat: 8g, Cholesterol: 65mg, Sodium: 76mg, Carbohydrates: 5g, Fiber: 0g, Protein: 26g

Chunky Chicken Salad

GLUTEN-FREE • DAIRY-FREE • NIGHTSHADE-FREE

SERVES 4   **PREP** 10 minutes   **COOK** 20 minutes

I have always loved chicken salad, but traditional recipes usually include mayonnaise. You'll never know that ingredient is missing when you bite into this tangy, nutrient-dense alternative. I usually eat this by itself, but I also like to serve it over a bed of fresh greens to take advantage of even more anti-inflammatory nutrients.

1 pound boneless, skinless chicken breasts

5 medium carrots, grated

2 large celery stalks, chopped

4 scallions, chopped

½ cup halved blueberries

½ cup sunflower seeds

⅓ cup extra-virgin olive oil

2 tablespoons balsamic vinegar

1 garlic clove, chopped

¼ teaspoon kosher salt

¼ teaspoon freshly ground black pepper

1. Preheat the oven to 375°F.

2. Halve the chicken breasts and arrange them in a single layer in the bottom of a medium saucepan. Pour in enough water to cover the chicken by an inch.

3. Bring to a boil, then cover, reduce the heat to low, and simmer for 15 minutes, or until the chicken reaches an internal temperature of 165°F. Remove the chicken from the poaching liquid and transfer to a cutting board.

4. Meanwhile, in a large bowl, combine the carrots, celery, scallions, blueberries, and sunflower seeds.

5. In a small bowl, whisk together the olive oil, vinegar, garlic, salt, and pepper.

6. Dice the cooked chicken or shred it using a food processor.

7. Add the shredded chicken to the vegetable mixture and drizzle the dressing over all of the ingredients.

8. Mix well to coat.

Variation Tip: This chicken salad is perfect, but you can change it by swapping out the sunflower seeds for walnuts. Or instead of scallions, try ½ medium red onion, chopped.

Per serving (¾ cup): Calories: 404, Total Fat: 26g, Saturated Fat: 3g, Cholesterol: 65mg, Sodium: 265mg, Carbohydrates: 15g, Fiber: 4g, Protein: 30g

Pecan-Crusted Chicken

GLUTEN-FREE • DAIRY-FREE • NIGHTSHADE-FREE

SERVES 4 **PREP** 10 minutes **COOK** 20 minutes

If you're looking to jazz up your chicken dinner, try this crunchy pecan-crusted version. The highlight of this recipe is the hint of rosemary combined with the slightly sweet pecans. Rosemary is a Mediterranean herb with powerful neurocognitive and anti-inflammatory benefits that provides a woodsy, warming element.

1 large egg, lightly beaten

2 tablespoons unsweetened plain almond milk

½ cup finely chopped pecans

½ cup gluten-free oat flour

1 teaspoon dried rosemary

¼ teaspoon kosher salt

1 pound boneless, skinless chicken breasts

1 tablespoon coconut oil

1. In a medium bowl, whisk together the egg and almond milk.

2. In a separate medium bowl, combine the pecans, oat flour, rosemary, and salt.

3. Dip the chicken breasts in the egg mixture, coating well on both sides.

4. Dredge the chicken in the pecan mixture, coating well on both sides.

5. In a large skillet over medium heat, warm the coconut oil.

6. Place the coated chicken in the skillet and cook for 8 minutes on each side, or until the chicken reaches an internal temperature of 165°F.

Substitution Tip: If you are avoiding eggs, use ¼ cup aquafaba liquid from a can of chickpeas as an egg substitute and whisk it together with the almond milk in step 1.

Per serving (1 chicken breast): Calories: 329, Total Fat: 22g, Saturated Fat: 4g, Cholesterol: 65mg, Sodium: 137mg, Carbohydrates: 6g, Fiber: 2g, Protein: 29g

Pineapple-Turkey Kabobs

GLUTEN-FREE • DAIRY-FREE • NIGHTSHADE-FREE

SERVES 4   **PREP** 10 minutes, plus 30 minutes to marinate   **COOK** 15 minutes

These slightly tangy kabobs are protein-packed and the perfect light meal. I serve these over a bed of cauliflower rice for an even heartier, nutrient-dense meal. If you don't have skewers for the kabobs, simply add all the ingredients to a lined baking sheet and create a sheet-pan dinner. These are great reheated for an easy lunch.

½ cup Dijon-Balsamic Vinaigrette (page 113)

2 tablespoons freshly squeezed lemon juice

2 garlic cloves, minced

1 pound turkey breast tenderloins, cut into 1½-inch cubes

1 large zucchini, halved lengthwise and cut into 1-inch chunks

1 large yellow squash, halved lengthwise and cut into 1-inch chunks

1 large yellow onion, chopped

1 cup pineapple chunks

1. Preheat the oven to 350°F. Line a baking sheet with parchment paper.

2. In a small bowl, whisk together the vinaigrette, lemon juice, and garlic.

3. Put the turkey, zucchini, squash, onion, pineapple, and marinade into a large sealable plastic bag and refrigerate for 30 minutes.

4. Thread the turkey, vegetable, and fruit chunks onto four skewers, alternating the pieces as you go. Discard the marinade.

5. Place the kabobs on the baking sheet and bake for 12 minutes (rotating the skewers one time), or until the turkey reaches an internal temperature of 165°F.

Make It Easier Tip: To save time and make this dish even more flavorful, prepare your ingredients the day before and marinate them in the refrigerator overnight.

Per serving (1 skewer): Calories: 339, Total Fat: 19g, Saturated Fat: 2g, Cholesterol: 55mg, Sodium: 339mg, Carbohydrates: 16g, Fiber: 3g, Protein: 31g

Turmeric Turkey Burgers

GLUTEN-FREE • DAIRY-FREE • NIGHTSHADE-FREE

SERVES 4　**PREP** 10 minutes　**COOK** 15 minutes

I love a juicy burger—it makes me think of summer grilling season. You don't have to wait for summer to enjoy this baked, anti-inflammatory burger. I serve these Turmeric Turkey Burgers in the traditional way with my favorite burger toppings, Crispy Kale Chips (page 39), and Honey-Ginger Fruit Salad (page 36).

1 pound ground turkey

1 medium yellow onion, finely chopped

2 teaspoons ground ginger

1 teaspoon ground turmeric

1 tablespoon freshly squeezed lemon juice

1 teaspoon kosher salt

1 tablespoon gluten-free oat flour

1. Preheat the oven to 400°F. Line a baking sheet with parchment paper.

2. In a large bowl, combine the ground turkey, onion, ginger, turmeric, lemon juice, and salt. Mix well.

3. Add the oat flour and mix until well combined.

4. Form 4 patties and place them on the baking sheet.

5. Bake for 15 minutes, or until the turkey reaches an internal temperature of 165°F.

Ingredient Tip: Turkey can quickly become dry if overcooked. Using a thermometer, check the internal temperature frequently. Removing the patties from the oven promptly will help preserve their moisture.

Per serving (1 patty): Calories: 193, Total Fat: 10g, Saturated Fat: 3g, Cholesterol: 90mg, Sodium: 577mg, Carbohydrates: 5g, Fiber: 1g, Protein: 21g

Skillet Beef and Peppers

GLUTEN-FREE • DAIRY-FREE

SERVES 4   **PREP** 10 minutes   **COOK** 25 minutes

Eating a rainbow of colors when it comes to produce will ensure your intake of a wide variety of vitamins, minerals, and phytonutrients to help fight inflammation. Instead of just choosing the less expensive green peppers, opt instead for all colors. This will brighten your plate and increase the variety of nutrients you're getting.

1 pound grass-fed ground beef

1 head cauliflower, roughly chopped

2 tablespoons extra-virgin olive oil

1 cup chopped multi-colored bell peppers

1 (16-ounce) can tomato sauce

1 tablespoon ground cumin

1 teaspoon chili powder

1 teaspoon garlic powder

¼ teaspoon kosher salt

¼ teaspoon freshly ground black pepper

2 cups spinach

1. In a medium skillet over medium heat, sauté the beef for 7 minutes, or until browned.

2. Put the cauliflower into a food processor and pulse until the cauliflower is the consistency of rice.

3. In a large skillet over medium heat, warm the olive oil. Add the bell peppers and sauté until soft, about 5 minutes.

4. Add the tomato sauce, cumin, chili powder, garlic powder, salt, black pepper, and riced cauliflower. Cook over medium heat until the cauliflower rice is soft, about 5 minutes.

5. Drain the beef and add it and the spinach to the pepper mixture.

6. Reduce the heat to low and simmer for 4 minutes, or until the spinach is wilted.

7. Serve immediately.

Variation Tip: If you are avoiding nightshades, omit the tomato sauce, bell peppers, and chili powder and add 1 cup chopped zucchini.

Per serving (about 1½ cups): Calories: 324, Total Fat: 19g, Saturated Fat: 6g, Cholesterol: 75mg, Sodium: 837mg, Carbohydrates: 13g, Fiber: 5g, Protein: 27g

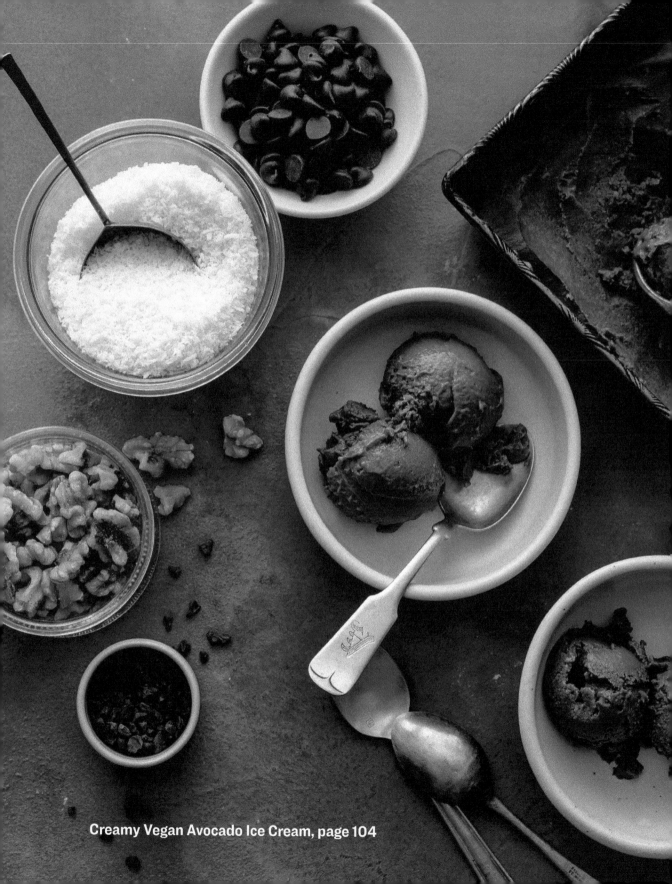

Creamy Vegan Avocado Ice Cream, page 104

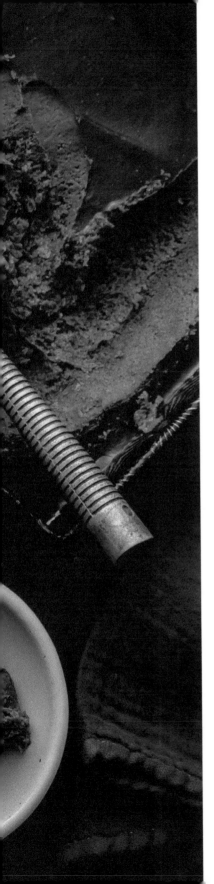

8
DESSERTS

Creamy Vegan Avocado Ice Cream

GLUTEN-FREE • DAIRY-FREE • NIGHTSHADE-FREE • VEGAN

SERVES 3   **PREP** 15 minutes, plus 4 hours to freeze

You may not think of avocados as a dessert food, but this recipe will change your mind. Avocados are a great source of monounsaturated fats, which help fight inflammation, and they are high in fiber to feed your gut microbiome. If you can't wait for this recipe to freeze, it's no problem. You can eat this ice cream as a pudding!

1 large ripe avocado, pitted, peeled, and diced

½ large ripe banana

¼ cup unsweetened vanilla almond milk

¼ cup maple syrup

3 tablespoons cacao powder

½ teaspoon vanilla extract

¼ teaspoon kosher salt

Chopped nuts, fresh fruit, and/or dark chocolate chips, for topping (optional)

1. Put the avocado, banana, almond milk, maple syrup, cacao powder, vanilla, and salt into a food processor or blender. Blend on high until smooth.

2. Pour the mixture into a shallow dish and freeze for 4 hours, or overnight.

3. Allow the ice cream to sit out for 10 to 15 minutes to soften before serving.

4. Top with chopped nuts, fresh fruit, dark chocolate chips, or any of your favorite ice cream toppings, if desired.

Variation Tip: You can experiment with new flavorings by adding nuts, dark chocolate chips, or unsweetened shredded coconut to the blender in step 1.

Per serving (½ cup): Calories: 240, Total Fat: 13g, Saturated Fat: 4g, Cholesterol: 0mg, Sodium: 178mg, Carbohydrates: 38g, Fiber: 11g, Protein: 6g

Pumpkin–Chocolate Chip Cookies

GLUTEN-FREE • NIGHTSHADE-FREE • VEGETARIAN

MAKES 24 cookies   **PREP** 15 minutes   **COOK** 15 minutes

These decadent sweet treats will make your whole house smell like the holidays. Pumpkin, a great source of fiber and vitamin A, provides the perfect flavor and texture for these cake-like cookies.

½ cup coconut oil, melted

1 teaspoon vanilla extract

1 cup pumpkin purée

⅓ cup honey

1½ cups tigernut flour

¼ teaspoon kosher salt

½ teaspoon baking soda

¼ teaspoon baking powder

1½ teaspoons cinnamon

¼ teaspoon ground nutmeg

½ cup dark chocolate chips
(>70% dark chocolate)

1. Preheat the oven to 350°F. Line a baking sheet with parchment paper.

2. In a large bowl, mix together the coconut oil, vanilla, pumpkin, and honey. Set aside.

3. In a separate large bowl, whisk together the tigernut flour, salt, baking soda, baking powder, cinnamon, and nutmeg.

4. Slowly add the wet ingredients to the dry ingredients. Mix well. Fold in the chocolate chips.

5. Using a tablespoon, shape the dough into balls and drop them on the baking sheet, spacing them about 1 inch apart. These cookies will not flatten as they bake, so press each ball gently with a spoon before baking.

6. Bake for 12 to 15 minutes, or until lightly browned and somewhat firm. Allow the cookies to cool for 5 minutes before transferring to a cooling rack.

7. Store in an airtight container in the refrigerator for up to 1 week.

Ingredient Tip: Tigernut is a small root vegetable that has become a popular gluten-free snack. Tigernut flour is a wonderful gluten- and grain-free substitute in many baked goods. You can find it in health food stores or online.

Per serving (1 cookie): Calories: 95, Total Fat: 7g, Saturated Fat: 5g, Cholesterol: 0mg, Sodium: 48mg, Carbohydrates: 9g, Fiber: 2g, Protein: 1g

Banana-Nut Bread

GLUTEN-FREE • DAIRY-FREE • NIGHTSHADE-FREE • VEGETARIAN

SERVES 12　**PREP** 10 minutes　**COOK** 35 minutes

I loved banana-nut bread as a kid, so when I chose to go gluten- and dairy-free, I thought I would have to miss out on that and so many more of my favorite desserts. But this light, fluffy banana-nut bread tops even my original family recipe—and I don't have to sacrifice anything! In fact, my husband requested this recipe for his birthday dessert this year, and we served it with a scoop of the Creamy Vegan Avocado Ice Cream (page 104).

3 ripe bananas, mashed

1 teaspoon vanilla extract

¼ cup almond butter

2 large eggs

½ cup coconut flour

¾ teaspoon baking soda

½ teaspoon ground cinnamon

¼ teaspoon kosher salt

½ cup chopped walnuts

1. Preheat the oven to 350°F. Line a 9-by-5-inch loaf pan with parchment paper.

2. In a large bowl, combine the bananas, vanilla, and almond butter. Mix until creamy.

3. Mix in the eggs until well combined.

4. Add the coconut flour, baking soda, cinnamon, salt, and walnuts and mix well.

5. Pour the batter into the loaf pan and bake for 30 to 35 minutes.

6. Allow to cool completely before cutting into 12 slices.

Variation Tip: Fold in ½ cup dark chocolate chips before baking.

Per serving (1 slice): Calories: 129, Total Fat: 8g, Saturated Fat: 1g, Cholesterol: 27mg, Sodium: 153mg, Carbohydrates: 12g, Fiber: 4g, Protein: 4g

No-Bake Coconut Energy Bites

GLUTEN-FREE • DAIRY-FREE • NIGHTSHADE-FREE • VEGETARIAN

SERVES 8 **PREP** 15 minutes, plus 30 minutes to chill

These slightly sweet coconut energy bites with just a hint of sea salt are the perfect afternoon snack or after-dinner treat. I love to keep a batch of these in the refrigerator for a quick on-the-go pick-me-up.

¾ cup tigernut flour

½ cup unsweetened shredded coconut

¼ teaspoon sea salt

2 tablespoons coconut oil, melted

2 tablespoons honey

1 tablespoon cacao powder

1 teaspoon vanilla extract

1. Put the tigernut flour, coconut, and salt into a food processor. Pulse 5 times, or until combined. (You can also mix by hand, if needed.)

2. Add the coconut oil, honey, cacao powder, and vanilla and pulse about 15 times, or until the mixture is a little crumbly but still holds together when formed into a ball.

3. Using a tablespoon, form the mixture into 16 energy bites.

4. Refrigerate for 30 minutes, or until the bites have set.

5. Store in an airtight container in the refrigerator.

> **Variation Tip:** You can use ¾ cup coconut flour as a substitute for the tigernut flour.

Per serving (2 energy bites): Calories: 141, Total Fat: 10g, Saturated Fat: 7g, Cholesterol: 0mg, Sodium: 61mg, Carbohydrates: 11g, Fiber: 4g, Protein: 2g

Almond Butter Granola Bars

GLUTEN-FREE • NIGHTSHADE-FREE • VEGETARIAN

SERVES 12 **PREP** 10 minutes, plus 30 minutes to chill

Instead of buying prepackaged granola bars, which are often made with inflammatory ingredients and unhealthy additives, make these unbelievable almond butter granola bars. They come together in no time and are a great portable energy bar that also makes a nice dessert. For the nuts in this recipe, I like a combination of cashews and pecans, but feel free to experiment with your own favorite varieties.

1 cup packed pitted Medjool dates

1 cup gluten-free rolled oats

½ cup raw nuts

¼ cup dark chocolate chips (>70% dark chocolate)

1 cup almond butter

¼ cup honey

1. Put the dates, oats, nuts, and chocolate chips into a food processor and process until all ingredients are incorporated and slightly chunky, about 45 seconds.

2. Transfer the processed ingredients to a large bowl.

3. In a small saucepan over medium heat, heat the almond butter and honey and stir well to combine.

4. Pour the melted honey–almond butter mixture into the dry ingredients and mix well to incorporate. (If the ingredients are still dry after mixing, add more melted honey or almond butter.)

5. Transfer the mixture to an 8-by-8-inch baking pan and, using a piece of parchment paper between your hands and the mixture, mash it into a solid, even layer (about ½ inch thick).

6. Refrigerate for 30 minutes.

7. Cut into 12 bars and store in an airtight container in the refrigerator for up to 2 weeks.

Batch Cook Tip: These bars freeze well, so double your recipe and freeze half for another time. Cut the bars, wrap them individually in parchment paper, and store them in a freezer-safe sealable plastic storage bag.

Per serving (1 bar): Calories: 271, Total Fat: 16g, Saturated Fat: 2g, Cholesterol: 0mg, Sodium: 94mg, Carbohydrates: 32g, Fiber: 4g, Protein: 6g

Chocolate Chip Cookie Dough

GLUTEN-FREE • NIGHTSHADE-FREE • VEGETARIAN

SERVES 8   **PREP** 10 minutes

Remember this guilty pleasure? Everyone loves chocolate chip cookie dough, but eating it has drawbacks, like added sugar and the potentially harmful bacteria found in uncooked eggs. Sure, you can try premade safe versions, but this rich, smooth cookie dough is so simple to make you'll never go back to store-bought.

½ cup tigernut flour

¼ cup tapioca flour

5 tablespoons grass-fed butter

3 teaspoons honey

1 teaspoon vanilla extract

¼ teaspoon kosher salt

2 tablespoons dark chocolate chips (>70% dark chocolate)

1. Put the tigernut flour, tapioca flour, butter, honey, vanilla, and salt into a blender and blend until smooth.

2. Transfer the dough to a medium bowl and fold in the chocolate chips.

3. Form the dough into 8 balls of equal size.

4. Store in an airtight container in the refrigerator for up to 7 days.

Ingredient Tip: If you can't find >70% dark chocolate chips, simply chop a >70% dark chocolate bar into small chunks and mix it into your dough.

Per serving (1 cookie dough ball): Calories: 119, Total Fat: 9g, Saturated Fat: 5g, Cholesterol: 19mg, Sodium: 110mg, Carbohydrates: 9g, Fiber: 1g, Protein: 1g

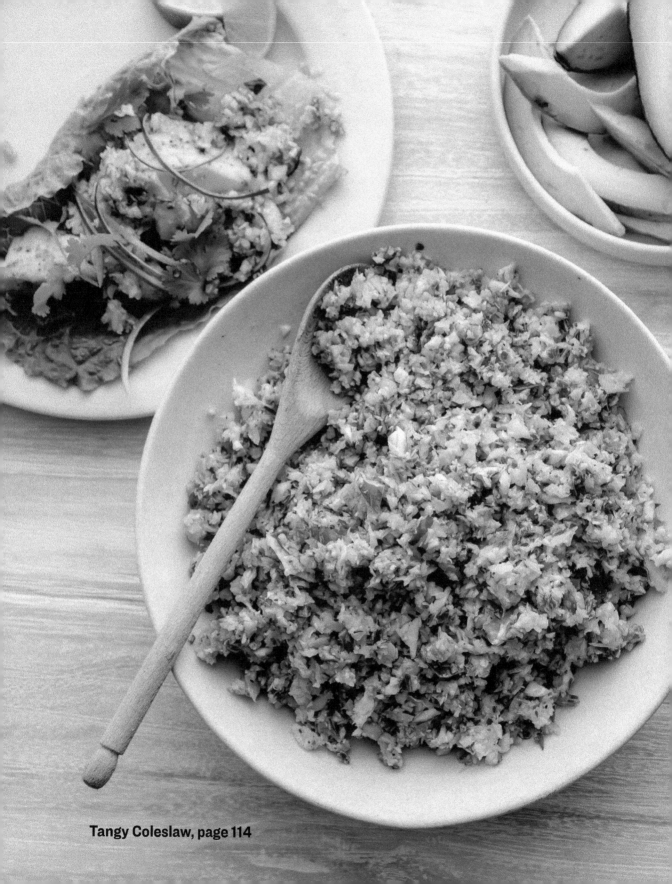

Tangy Coleslaw, page 114

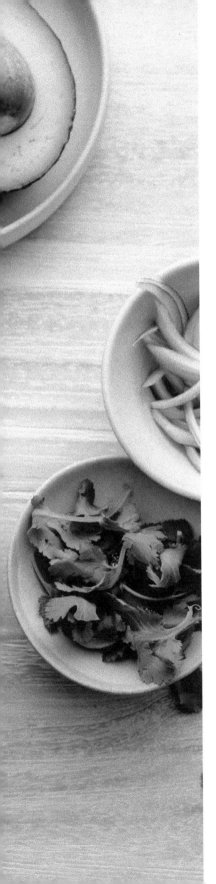

9

CONDIMENTS, DRESSINGS, AND SAUCES

Spinach-Pecan Pesto

GLUTEN-FREE • DAIRY-FREE • NIGHTSHADE-FREE • VEGAN

MAKES 2½ cups   **PREP** 10 minutes

Traditional pesto contains dairy, but you'll never know that ingredient is missing in this recipe. The bright green color makes this a fun addition to sandwiches, salads, and pizza, or it can be used as a dip for fresh vegetables. This pesto is the perfect example of how to modify a recipe to maintain fabulous taste without sacrificing your healthy eating style.

2 cups spinach

½ cup pecans

3 garlic cloves

¼ teaspoon kosher salt

¼ teaspoon freshly ground black pepper

½ cup extra-virgin olive oil

1. Put the spinach, pecans, ¼ cup water, garlic, salt, and pepper into a food processor and blend until well combined.

2. Slowly pour in the olive oil while processing until the mixture comes together and a paste is formed.

3. Store in an airtight container in the refrigerator for up to 5 days.

Variation Tip: Walnuts are a great substitution for the pecans.

Per serving (¼ cup): Calories: 128, Total Fat: 14g, Saturated Fat: 2g, Cholesterol: 0mg, Sodium: 63mg, Carbohydrates: 1g, Fiber: 1g, Protein: 1g

Dijon-Balsamic Vinaigrette

GLUTEN-FREE • DAIRY-FREE • NIGHTSHADE-FREE • VEGAN

MAKES ⅓ cup   **PREP** 5 minutes

This flavorful dressing is the perfect, quick alternative to the processed, unhealthy oils and additives found in most store-bought dressings. Extra-virgin olive oil contains powerful monounsaturated fats and antioxidants, making it one of my favorite go-to foods to fight inflammation. This dressing comes together in almost no time, so you can mix it up right before your meal.

¼ cup extra-virgin olive oil

2 tablespoons balsamic vinegar

1 tablespoon Dijon mustard

2 garlic cloves, chopped

¼ teaspoon dried oregano

¼ teaspoon dried basil

¼ teaspoon dried thyme

¼ teaspoon kosher salt

¼ teaspoon freshly ground black pepper

In a mason jar or salad shaker, place the olive oil, vinegar, mustard, garlic, oregano, basil, thyme, salt, and pepper and shake well to combine.

Variation Tip: Avocado oil also works well for this dressing.

Per serving (2 tablespoons): Calories: 154, Total Fat: 17g, Saturated Fat: 2g, Cholesterol: 0mg, Sodium: 254mg, Carbohydrates: 1g, Fiber: 0g, Protein: 0g

Tangy Coleslaw

GLUTEN-FREE • DAIRY-FREE • NIGHTSHADE-FREE • VEGAN

SERVES 8   **PREP** 10 minutes

This tangy coleslaw is a great condiment, but I also use this recipe as a potent anti-inflammatory side dish! Cabbage, another fantastic cruciferous vegetable, contains specific antioxidants known to help reduce blood markers of inflammation. It's also a high source of fiber to feed the gut microbiome, as well as vitamin C to keep the immune system strong.

1 red onion

½ head green cabbage

3 medium carrots

2 celery stalks

½ cup extra-virgin olive oil

¼ cup pomegranate vinegar or apple cider vinegar (with the mother)

2 tablespoons Dijon mustard

1 teaspoon kosher salt

1 teaspoon freshly ground black pepper

1 teaspoon celery salt

1 teaspoon ground cumin

1. Put the onion into a food processor and pulse until shredded (make sure not to overprocess). Repeat, separately, with the cabbage, carrots, and celery.

2. In a large bowl, mix together the shredded vegetables.

3. In a small bowl, whisk together the olive oil, vinegar, mustard, salt, pepper, celery salt, and cumin.

4. Pour the dressing over the shredded vegetables and toss to coat.

5. Store in an airtight container in the refrigerator for up to 3 days.

Variation Tip: Substitute red cabbage for the green cabbage or use a mixture of both to make this dish more colorful and festive!

Per serving (¼ cup): Calories: 141, Total Fat: 13g, Saturated Fat: 2g, Cholesterol: 0mg, Sodium: 372mg, Carbohydrates: 7g, Fiber: 2g, Protein: 1g

Velvety Turmeric Sauce

GLUTEN-FREE • DAIRY-FREE • NIGHTSHADE-FREE • VEGAN

MAKES 5 cups   **COOK** 30 minutes

Turmeric has been used throughout history for its unique flavor and medicinal properties. Its powerful anti-inflammatory and antioxidant capacity is a result of the active compound curcumin. This delicious sauce is one way to increase your intake of those helpful curcuminoids and can be used in stir-fries, as a vegetable dip, as a sauce for Vegan "Meatballs" (page 68), or thinned with some extra-virgin olive oil to be used as a salad dressing.

3 (13.5-ounce) cans full-fat coconut milk

2 teaspoons kosher salt

1 teaspoon ground turmeric

1 teaspoon ground cumin

1 teaspoon garlic powder

½ teaspoon freshly ground black pepper

1. Place the coconut milk, salt, turmeric, cumin, garlic powder, and pepper in a large saucepan and bring to a boil over high heat.

2. Reduce the heat to low and simmer for 30 minutes to allow to thicken.

3. Add to your favorite prepared dish or store in an air-tight container in the refrigerator for up to 3 days.

Variation Tip: This recipe freezes well, so double the amount and store it away for a quick, easy way to flavor a variety of dishes.

Per serving (¼ cup): Calories: 113, Total Fat: 12g, Saturated Fat: 11g, Cholesterol: 0mg, Sodium: 240mg, Carbohydrates: 2g, Fiber: 0g, Protein: 1g

Easy Anti-Inflammatory Vegetable Dressing

GLUTEN-FREE • DAIRY-FREE • VEGETARIAN

MAKES ⅔ cup　**PREP** 5 minutes

Vegetables are a mainstay of the Mediterranean diet and although they taste awesome on their own, sometimes you want to dress them up a bit. This simple, tangy dressing is the perfect choice to punch up the flavor of your favorite veggies and maximize your intake of anti-inflammatory spices.

⅔ cup unsweetened plain almond milk

¼ cup whole-milled flaxseed

1 tablespoon apple cider vinegar (with the mother)

1 tablespoon honey

½ teaspoon ground turmeric

½ teaspoon ground ginger

½ teaspoon curry powder

⅛ teaspoon mustard powder

⅛ teaspoon kosher salt

⅛ teaspoon freshly ground black pepper

1. Place the almond milk, flaxseed, vinegar, honey, turmeric, ginger, curry powder, mustard powder, salt, and pepper into a blender and blend until smooth.

2. Store in an airtight container in the refrigerator for up to 5 days.

Substitution Tip: If you are avoiding nightshades, eliminate the curry powder and double the turmeric to 1 teaspoon.

Per serving (2 tablespoons): Calories: 64, Total Fat: 3g, Saturated Fat: 0g, Cholesterol: 0mg, Sodium: 81mg, Carbohydrates: 7g, Fiber: 2g, Protein: 2g

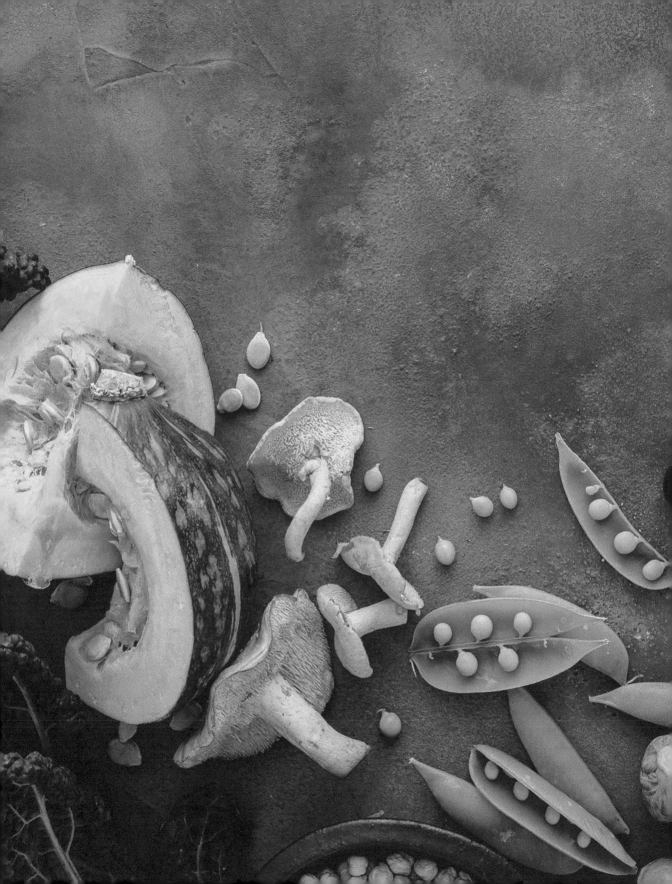

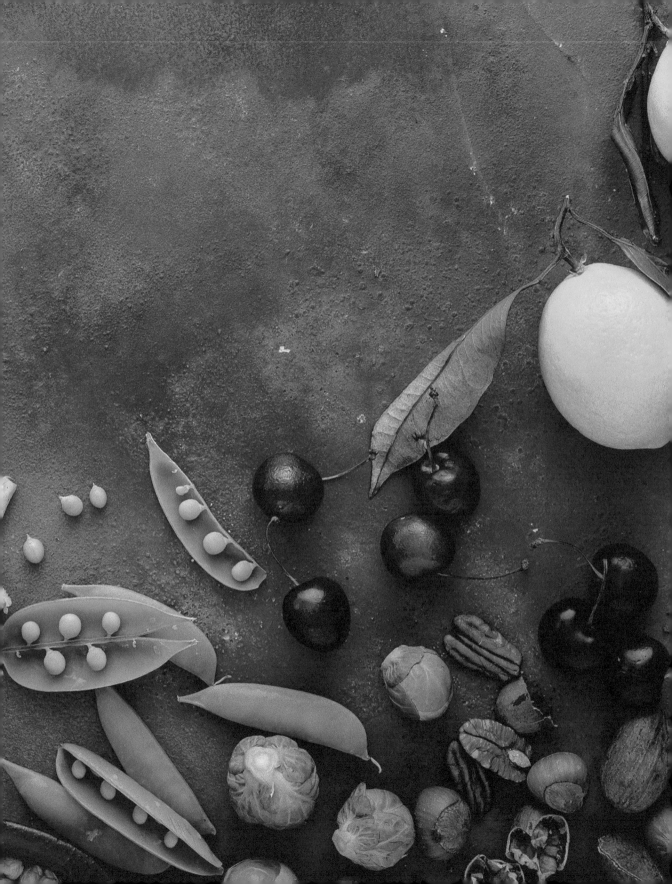

Measurement Conversions

	US STANDARD	US STANDARD (OUNCES)	METRIC (APPROXIMATE)
VOLUME EQUIVALENTS (LIQUID)	2 TABLESPOONS	1 FL. OZ.	30 ML
	¼ CUP	2 FL. OZ.	60 ML
	½ CUP	4 FL. OZ.	120 ML
	1 CUP	8 FL. OZ.	240 ML
	1½ CUPS	12 FL. OZ.	355 ML
	2 CUPS OR 1 PINT	16 FL. OZ.	475 ML
	4 CUPS OR 1 QUART	32 FL. OZ.	1 L
	1 GALLON	128 FL. OZ.	4 L
VOLUME EQUIVALENTS (DRY)	⅛ TEASPOON		0.5 ML
	¼ TEASPOON		1 ML
	½ TEASPOON		2 ML
	¾ TEASPOON		4 ML
	1 TEASPOON		5 ML
	1 TABLESPOON		15 ML
	¼ CUP		59 ML
	⅓ CUP		79 ML
	½ CUP		118 ML
	⅔ CUP		156 ML
	¾ CUP		177 ML
	1 CUP		235 ML
	2 CUPS OR 1 PINT		475 ML
	3 CUPS		700 ML
	4 CUPS OR 1 QUART		1 L
	½ GALLON		2 L
	1 GALLON		4 L
WEIGHT EQUIVALENTS	½ OUNCE		15 G
	1 OUNCE		30 G
	2 OUNCES		60 G
	4 OUNCES		115 G
	8 OUNCES		225 G
	12 OUNCES		340 G
	16 OUNCES OR 1 POUND		455 G

	FAHRENHEIT (F)	CELSIUS (C) (APPROXIMATE)
OVEN TEMPERATURES	250°F	120°C
	300°F	150°C
	325°F	180°C
	375°F	190°C
	400°F	200°C
	425°F	220°C
	450°F	230°C

Resources

WEBSITES:

NutriSense Nutrition Consulting, LLC (NutriSenseNutrition.com): Blog and website from author Kellie Blake. Functional nutrition information for anyone hoping to prevent or reverse a chronic disease. Kellie shares her own personal story, recipes, and ways to improve quality of life with lifestyle- and nutrition-related strategies.

National Psoriasis Foundation (Psoriasis.org): Website dedicated to psoriasis treatment. Contains research trial information and the latest psoriasis treatment options.

The American Academy of Dermatology (AAD.org): Website providing resources for all skin-related conditions.

Autoimmune Wellness (AutoimmuneWellness.com): Website with resources and recipes for those with autoimmune disorders.

Heal with Food (HealWithFood.org): Website providing information and recipes for healing psoriasis.

Your Guide to Healthy Sleep (https://www.nhlbi.nih.gov/files/docs/public/sleep/healthy_sleep.pdf): United States Department of Health & Human Services; National Institutes of Health; and National Heart, Lung, and Blood Institute document providing healthy sleep information.

The American Heart Association (https://www.heart.org/en/healthy-living/healthy-lifestyle/stress-management) Website addressing healthy stress-management techniques.

BOOKS:

Axe, Josh. *Eat Dirt: Why Leaky Gut May Be the Root Cause of Your Health Problems and 5 Surprising Steps to Cure It.* New York: Harperwave, 2016.

Bland, Jeffrey S. *The Disease Delusion.* New York: Harperwave, 2014.

Chopra, Deepak. *Perfect Digestion.* New York: Three Rivers Press, 1995.

Hyman, Mark. *Food, What the Heck Should I Eat?* New York: Little Brown and Company, 2018.

Myers, Amy. *The Autoimmune Solution: Prevent and Reverse the Full Spectrum of Inflammatory Symptoms and Disease.* New York: HarperOne, 2017.

Pagano, John O. A. *Healing Psoriasis: The Natural Alternative.* Hoboken, NJ: Wiley, 2009.

References

Barrea, Luigi, Francesca Nappi, Carolina Di Somma, Maria Cristina Savanelli, Andrea Falco, Anna Balato, and Silvia Savastano. "Environmental Risk Factors in Psoriasis: The Point of View of the Nutritionist." *International Journal of Environmental Research and Public Health* 13, no. 7 (July 13, 2016): 743. doi: 10.3390/ijerph13070743.

Barrea, Luigi, Maria Cristina Savanelli, Carolina Di Somma, Maddalena Napolitano, Matteo Megna, Annamaria Colao, and Silvia Savastano. "Vitamin D and its Role in Psoriasis: An Overview of the Dermatologist and Nutritionist." *Reviews in Endocrine and Metabolic Disorders,* 18, no. 2 (June 2017): 195–205. doi: 10.1007/s11154-017-9411-6.

Barrea, Luigi, Paolo Emidio Macchia, Giovanni Tarantino, Carolina Di Somma, Elena Pane, Nicola Balato, Maddalena Napolitano, Annamaria Colao, and Silvia Savastano. "Nutrition: A Key Environmental Dietary Factor in Clinical Severity and Cardi-Metabolic Risk in Psoriatic Male Patients Evaluated by 7-day Food-Frequency Questionnaire." *Journal of Translational Medicine,* 13, article no. 303 (September 16, 2015). doi: 10.1186/s12967-015-0658-y.

Gaby, Alan R. *Nutritional Medicine.* 2nd ed. Concord, NH: Fritz Perlberg, 2017.

Gaforio, José, Francesco Visioli, Catalina Alarcón-de-la-Lastra, Olga Castañer, Miguel Delgado-Rodríguez, Monserrat Fitó, Antonio Hernández, et al. "Virgin Olive Oil and Health: Summary of the III International Conference on Virgin Olive Oil and Health Consensus Report, JAEN (Spain) 2018." *Nutrients* 11, no. 9 (September 2019): 2039. doi.org/10.3390/nu11092039.

Goldman, Daniel, and Richard Davidson. *Altered Traits: Science Reveals How Meditation Changes Your Mind, Brain, and Body.* New York: Avery, 2017.

Phan, Céline, Mathilde Touvier, Emmanuelle Kesse-Guyot, Moufidath Adjibade, Serge Hercberg, Pierre Wolkenstein, Olivier Chosidow, Khaled Ezzedine, and Emilie Sbidian. "Association Between Mediterranean Anti-inflammatory Dietary Profile and Severity of Psoriasis." *JAMA Dermatology* 154, no. 9 (September 2018): 1017–1024. doi: 10.1001/jamadermatol.2018.2127.

Selhub, Eva, Alan Logan, and Alison Bested. "Fermented Foods, Microbiota, and Mental Health: Ancient Practice Meets Nutritional Psychiatry." *Journal of Physiological Anthropology* 33, article no. 2 (2014). doi: 10.1186/1880-6805-33-2.

Slavin, Joanne, and Beate Lloyd. "Health Benefits of Fruits and Vegetables." *Advances in Nutrition* 3, no. 4 (2012): 506–16. doi: 10.3945/an.112.002154.

Sugizake, Claire S.A., and Maria Margareth V. Naves. "Potential Prebiotic Properties of Nuts and Edible Seeds and Their Relationship to Obesity." *Nutrients* 10, no. 11 (November 2018): 1645. doi: 10.3390/nu10111645.

U.S. Department of Health & Human Services National Heart, Lung, and Blood Institute. "Metabolic Syndrome." Accessed October 15, 2019. https://www.nhlbi.nih.gov/health-topics/metabolic-syndrome.

Index

Acknowledgments

Thanks to my husband, Will, for being the ultimate taste-tester and kitchen assistant! I appreciate my parents—Mary, Steve, Greg, and Gina—for teaching me to think outside the box and my sisters—Heather and Kristen—for always being the epitome of selfless. Thanks to my nephews, Zion and Zachary, for letting me teach you the importance of wholesome food at young ages. Special thanks to my cousin Jaclyn for getting me started on my healing journey, Dr. Tom Rushton for letters of recommendation and helping me share my message with our community, and Lora Jody for your mentorship and entrepreneurial spirit. Special thanks to my in-laws, extended family, friends, and coworkers: You are all supportive, caring, awesome people.

To my clients: Your dedication to the process of lifestyle change is an inspiration to me and others around you, and I am so proud.

Finally, thank you to the entire Callisto team for your patience, kind words, and expertise.

About the Author

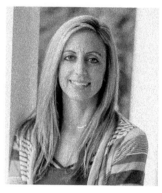 **Kellie Blake, RDN, LD, IFNCP,** is a registered dietitian specializing in functional nutrition. In addition to her career as a full-time psychiatric dietitian and her work with hospice patients, Kellie co-owns a private practice, NutriSense Nutrition Consulting, LLC, with Brandi Sentz, MA, RDN, LD, CDE. In her private practice, Kellie determines the root causes of symptoms and uses a functional nutrition approach to help her clients regain their health and quality of life. Kellie is also a health and nutrition writer and currently serves on the editorial board at Integrative Practitioner, where she shares her client case studies.

Kellie has used functional nutrition to reverse her own autoimmune disease, and she is passionate about sharing the "food as medicine" message. Kellie maintains a healthy living blog at **www.NutriSenseNutrition.com** and shares her favorite recipes on Instagram @NutriSenseNutrition. Kellie is enthusiastic about health and wellness and enjoys weight training, running, biking, practicing yoga, and spending time in nature with her husband, Will, and their three dogs.

CPSIA information can be obtained
at www.ICGtesting.com
Printed in the USA
BVHW050603221021
619534BV00005B/6